One Day at a Time

Pat Seed MBE

One Day at a Time

Pan Books
in association with Heinemann

First published 1979 by William Heinemann Ltd
This edition published 1979 by Pan Books Ltd
Cavaye Place, London SW10 9PG
in association with William Heinemann Ltd
© Pat Seed 1979
ISBN 0 330 25897 4
Printed and bound in Great Britain by
Richard Clay (The Chaucer Press) Ltd, Bungay, Suffolk

For every man, woman and child whose
love and concern provided a lifeline

Contents

Illustrations

Mrs Snowdon, Pat Seed, Dr Hounsfield and Nicola Farrow
make sure that the stone is well and truly laid

The EMI Scanner 7070 and control panel

A patient being put into position for CT diagnosis

Foreword

JEAN ROOK

There's something very precious about Pat Seed's life. I dread losing it.

But, if I can't have Pat, I want her book. I need her marvellous, down-to-earth words about cancer, and about life. And death.

I want them for myself, and for the millions of people Pat will be able to help, long after she's gone. Come to that, long after I'm gone, since she's always warning me I could smoke myself to death, or be flattened by a bus and beat her to it.

I won't call Pat Seed a heroine – though she is. Or say that she's one of the most important and valuable human beings I've ever known – though she is. I won't call her an inspiration, who's made a million pounds for others, because she's spoken direct to the hopes, and fears, and hearts of millions.

If I say all that, she'll ring up and ask me what happened to Fleet Street's biggest bitch – and who pulled my teeth out?

The last time I saw Pat I worried, as she knows all her friends do, when I'll see her again. Not because she's a 'tragic case', or because I won't get over the pain of her loss, when it comes.

I will, because I daren't not. Pat would ring me, out of the ether, brisk and cross with me for wasting moping time when I could be getting publicity for cancer research.

What worried me wasn't the cancer inside her, with which she has come to her own terms, however impossibly brave those terms may seem to the rest of us.

It was the book inside her, not written. And now I knew her well enough to point out that, if her deadline came up unexpectedly, the book which could be as much help to others as anything she's done, would go with her. So the time – however long or short – had come to get on with it.

I should go back to my first meeting with Pat. A colleague of mine had interviewed her for the *Express*. I'd only written a few, but very sincere words of admiration for her work in my column.

When an *Express* secretary said Mrs Seed was in the building, and would like to meet me, I felt the honour.

When your time is as valuable, and as limited, as Pat Seed's, you've as great a right as the Queen to be choosy where you spend it.

I don't know what I expected when she walked in to my office. Yes, I suppose I do. I thought she'd be thin and pale and ethereal – terribly in touch with the other world in which she accepts she's got a foot.

I thought that, sitting face to face with the first person I'd met who *knew* she had cancer – or, as Pat put it to me, 'they told me my number's up' – would be like being in at the Last Judgement. I felt I should have to drop my voice, if not my eyes, in her 'presence'.

She bounced in, in pink to match her cheeks, almost frighteningly alive. Reading shock in my face, she said, 'I know – I look so healthy I never get any sympathy.'

With her feet on the ground, and a cigarette in her hand ('that's one thing I don't have to worry about', she grinned) she told me her story.

Quite simply. As if she were telling me something very

unexpected and annoying that had happened to her on her holidays. Or on a bus.

She described the first gripping fear of the cancer, worse than the disease. The gradual facing up to it, walking round the horror, studying it from all angles and learning to cope.

The bad bit came when she told me about telling her children the truth. My own son is only seven, and I couldn't, God, I really *couldn't* do that.

Pat told me what she'd said, what the children said and how they'd come closer – in some fear, but mostly in love. She said I could do it if I had to, and I believed her, because – and this is her great strength – she's as ordinary, and northern, and full of common sense as I am.

Not a saint, or a prophet, but just Mrs Seed from up the road.

In front of me, as I write, I've a letter . . . 'Enjoy your trip to Greece. Don't look at the Acropolis and say it will be OK when it's finished. Cheers, Pat.'

I feel a bit guilty, for a split second, that I'll be sunbathing and swimming, miles from terror and hopefully years from death.

No, I don't feel guilty. How bloody daft can I be, as Pat would be the first to say. And, anyway, as she'd probably say next, I should watch it. I could drown.

I like to talk to Pat about death. She makes it seem so much smaller, and so natural. As she says, 'we all do it – in the end'.

But the first time I remarked, without thinking, 'you know, Pat, I'm *dying* to do such and such', I winced. She didn't, of course. Now I can smile when she describes a tough day's campaigning, when it all goes wrong, as 'the kiss of death'.

I haven't helped Pat, I'm afraid. She's helped me. I may have goaded her into writing. But I've leaned on her strength in our talks together. Because she is so fantastically, unbreakably strong.

I live in hope – that it will all go away, miraculously, and that she'll live forever.

When I'm with her, I have a desperate urge to touch her. Keep hold of her. Keep her here, not let her slip. When she's not here, I'll have the same urge to ring her number.

To ask her to tell me again how her life was, and her philosophy, because she makes cancer, and even death, just something you have to do eventually. Like the housework, or having a baby.

If she's not there to kick me occasionally, I shall moan about her a bit, instead of checking up that her work for cancer is going on.

That's why I kicked her into writing this book. Her words, in my hand, will be the next best thing to having her here. Dying with such grace, and strength, and beauty of spirit, while we sit together, having such an ordinary cup of tea.

I can't see Pat Seed as an angel. She's too earthy for the part.

But no doubt she'll be one – bustling with good will, and concern, and love.

1

Pathfinder

To the uninitiated, the editorial department of any newspaper office must seem like the aftermath of a tornado. Paper, paper, everywhere; typewriters clattering, telephones ringing; the teleprinters churning out miles of tape as news arrives from all parts of the world. Men and women with expressions of intense concentration and an overall sense of urgency, epitomising the pressures of that ever present deadline to be met.

No wonder pessimistic insurance companies estimate the life expectancy of the average journalist at a mere forty-eight years! In the labyrinth of offices above the impressively marbled foyer of the *Daily Express*, Fleet Street, London, I sat in a room more palatial than most. It had a carpet on the floor. It was nicely decorated and it even sported a vase of flowers.

On the outside of the door were the words: JEAN ROOK, ASSISTANT EDITOR. Behind the desk, the Queen of Fleet Street was glaring at me. I had called to see her on my way back to Euston Station after a recording session for London Weekend Television.

During our conversation I had mentioned that the experiences of the past months had provided enough material for a book. It was a book I knew should be written, but I was still too busy doing it, to write about it.

But if, dear reader, you are expecting a tale of woe, just because this book concerns cancer, put it down. It's not for you. If, however, you've enough stamina to keep pace with the greatest race of all – the human race – then proceed.

Be of good heart and bring your climbing boots with you. You'll need them. For this is a story of endeavour.

It began as a solitary journey along a mountainous path, when I set out into the unknown along a route I named the Scanner Trail. It has always been an uphill journey; rocky, exhausting, difficult and sometimes so fraught with problems that it seemed wellnigh impossible. But along that Trail, I met a lot of people. They were ready to offer me a helping hand and to walk the trail alongside of me. They brought with them laughter, gaiety and comradeship. Sometimes there was sorrow and a few tears.

They are wonderful people. Generous, kind hearted people. In all probability, they are just like you.

They helped to make the Scanner Trail the most rewarding, the most interesting and the most wonderful journey I've ever made or am ever likely to make.

And when we reached the top and saw the result of our labours, the sense of achievement was magnificent and the view was exhilarating.

So where did that journey begin?

I have sixteen typewritten foolscap pages which are the outpourings of a soul in torment. They were written before I went into the Christie on 19th May 1976 and were, I suppose, a journalist's attempt to 'write cancer out of her system'. They are the product of a state of shock. When I returned home after three weeks of radiotherapy treatment, I read over what I had written and decided it was no use to anyone, least of all, to me.

I told myself that if I was going to write about cancer, it must be in a positive way. It had to be of some help to those who may find themselves facing a similar situation.

My time in the Christie Hospital had left me with the impression that FEAR is cancer's greatest ally. The disease is a malignant random selector and a destructive leveller. The millionaire and the man on social security are equal candidates.

Without good health, we are nothing. We cannot take advantage of education, hold down a job, bring up a family or enjoy any of the good things of life. Money is no substitute.

Medical science has provided the cure for hitherto killer diseases. Vaccination and immunisation have decreased the mortality rate. One day, science will find the answer to cancer. Until that day comes, we fight it with the weapons to hand.

I did some rewriting.

The result was a series of four articles for the *West Lancashire Evening Gazette*. They were published in July 1976.

Headline: **Dread News, but it brought our family closer together.**

'If this should turn out to be cancer, my husband and I will want to know,' I told my doctor. 'Please,' I added, 'no medical mystique.'

He visibly relaxed.

'You don't know what a relief that is,' he said. 'There are times when I stand outside a house, trying to remember whether it is a home where the patient knows and the family doesn't – or vice versa.'

The wheel of circumstance spins and each time it comes to rest, it spotlights a facet of human existence; triumphs and tragedies; fortune and failure; courage and crime. A working journalist encounters all of these and more when reporting the kaleidoscope of human events.

Everyone has his own personal kaleidoscope.

Mine took on every shade of grey when I found that abdominal discomfort was due to cancerous tumours. My life as a wife, mother and journalist seemed to jar to a halt. Life had been busy, varied and always full of interest.

April 1976 . . . it was the beginning of a journey into the unknown. Not least, one of discovering what inner resources of faith, courage and hope were mine to call upon. The only way I could play it was with absolute truth – and what should a journalist be, if not a seeker of truth?

I know that there are cancer victims who absolutely refuse to accept the fact that they have cancer. For some people, this is the only way they can get through. They will discuss, intelligently, any subject under the sun. But *Cancer for them is a dirty word and, as such, is taboo. A general practitioner has to play it their way.*

At the age of forty-eight, I have been married almost twenty-five years. We have a son at college and a daughter about to take A-level examinations. We are a happy family.

Then in April, the future looked grim. I did not even know if I had a future.

After a laperotomy operation at our local hospital, the consultant surgeon confirmed that I had cancer and I was referred to the Christie Hospital, Manchester.

I spent a whole afternoon wondering how to tell our children, for the name Christie is synonymous with cancer. They would have to know.

My daughter was the first to arrive home and after discussion on pre-exam tension at school, I told her.

I watched her face change. Her eyes filled with tears and so did mine. Eventually we decided that in our different ways, we each had a fight on our hands. It would be a test of character for us both and show what we were made of.

Later, my son came home and I broke the news to him. 'Is it a shock?' I asked.

'I've known something was wrong, Mum. In a way it's far

better to know. Much better than to be kept in ignorance and to feel left out.'

My youngsters made me realise that their generation is far more resilient than we parents imagine. And because all four of us have known it has brought a sense of release, a certain kind of freedom. More than ever before, we are a close-knit family.

I am learning to take one day at a time, to work a little, to play a little. To enjoy what each day brings and ignore the flaws. The future is an unknown quantity.

Three days after the consultant told my husband that I had cancer, the Department of the Environment informed him that he had won £25 on 'Ernie'. We cried over the former and, because of it, the latter seemed so ludicrous that we were all helpless with laughter.

You cannot say the kaleidoscope lacks variety.

Headline: **In Place of Fear.**

It is a traumatic experience to find one has cancer. Cancer is something that happens to other people, not to oneself. Or so I thought . . .

There was a time when the only way one could expect to come out of the Christie Hospital, Manchester, was feet first, in a wooden box.

That was way back in 1892 when Sir Richard Copley Christie founded what was then known as The Home for Cancer Incurables. In those days the only hope of a cure was a miracle.

More than eighty years later it is a very different story. The Christie Hospital and Holt Radium Institute is one of the world's foremost cancer treatment hospitals and research centres. Yet, to a large extent, the fear and dread of the Victorian era still persist in the minds of the public and it hampers what could be potentially spectacular progress in the 'war' against cancer.

A typical example came to my notice when I was told of a branch of the Women's Institute whose committee had arranged for a talk to be given on this subject at their monthly meeting. Half the members failed to turn up. It is an ostrich, head-in-the-sand attitude and I am ashamed to say that until recently, I might have been among those who boycotted such a lecture.

Not any more.

Re-educating public thinking about cancer is the mammoth task being undertaken by four regional committees in Britain. The Manchester Regional Committee for Cancer Education, which serves most of the north-west of England, is centred on the Christie Hospital. The committee's lecturers are prepared to talk to any club group or organisation on the subject.

The hospital admits between 6,000 and 7,000 patients a year and has an extensive outpatients department. It is a far cry from the twenty-bed home for incurables of the last century. What is the success rate in terms of cures? 'Cure' is a word used with caution.

Mr R. L. Davison, the Committee's Director, said that of the patients discharged five years ago, just under fifty per cent are still 'cancer free'. If one could include the elderly who in the interim had died of a complaint other than cancer, that percentage would be considerably increased. But – and it is a very significant 'but' – if one could get the full co-operation of the public, in the form of more enlightened thinking, that percentage would rocket in spectacular fashion.

It is a sad fact of life that while research workers are beavering away in many corners of the world and a great deal of quiet progress is being made in cancer medicine – much of which never makes the headlines – the public is its own worst enemy. There is still a vast number of people who tend to regard all cancer patients as doomed.

Just how erroneous this thinking is has been brought home to me with great impact during a three-week sojourn in the

Christie. It has completely altered my outlook.

As well as the 'cancer free' there are a multitude of people holding down jobs and leading active, useful lives who are former patients of the Christie and who have cancer which is controlled by drugs. I hope to be among this number. Both the cured and the controlled are modern-day miracles and living tributes to the skill of the Christie doctors. They could do a great deal to change public thinking.

We should not be ashamed to admit that we have cancer any more than a diabetic is ashamed to admit that he or she has diabetes.

Of the two complaints, many forms of cancer are curable. Diabetes can only be controlled. And the chances of any form of cancer being cured are increased by early diagnosis, followed by early treatment; by persuading women to attend breast screening clinics and to have the cervical smear test. In both these extremely common forms of cancer in women, quite often there is no swelling, no pain until the disease has established a firm hold. Early diagnosis – the greater the chance of survival.

Fear is the root cause which hampers real progress. It is time the adversary was brought out from under the carpet.

It is time fear was replaced by positive public co-operation in the fight against the disease which is still the greatest scourge of mankind.

Headline: **The Patient Joins the Team.**

When I was first admitted to the Christie, it wasn't long before I was asking myself: 'What is it about this hospital that is different from any other in which I've been a patient?'

A ward of eighteen beds and eighteen women . . . all of us with cancer in one form or another and all of us apprehensive. Yet there was a wonderful atmosphere and morale was high.

The nursing staff of most hospitals is efficient and kind. Yet at the Christie, I was aware of some extra quality which I found hard to define. Was it extra dedication? A sort of hyper-vocation?

Yes, there were both of these, but eventually I realised that the key word at the Christie is teamwork.

The entire staff of the hospital, from the most eminent doctors through to porters and domestic workers play a tremendously supportive role. They are fully aware of the mental strain which accompanies the physical discomforts of cancer. The patient is made to feel an active member of the team. They have one object in view – to get you well, or as well as modern medical science can make you.

The emphasis on teamwork is apparent at the noonday clinic, a feature which is unique to the Christie. At noon each working day, new patients are seen by all available members of the medical staff, from students to senior clinicians.

I had heard fearsome tales about the radiotherapy treatment, but having had sixteen treatments of deep X-ray therapy, my personal experience was that it was not nearly so bad as I had expected.

The machine looked like something out of 'Dr Who' – a huge turquoise green polo mint with a protruding arm which swings through 180 degrees and on which was the business end. Its rays are invisible, powerful, healing and completely painless. The side effects are sickness, lethargy, loss of appetite and diarrhoea. Severity varies from one patient to another and some experience no side effects at all. But there are anti-sickness pills, one's bed on which to rest and the human body can exist for quite some time without food. No one is allowed to be in pain. An attentive nursing staff and modern pain killers see to that.

The radiotherapy department deals with some 200 patients a day on a range of equipment from those of 45–100 kilovolts designed for the treatment of simple skin cancers, through a range of radium and X-ray machinery accelerated up to eight million volts. In addition, there is a cobalt unit of one million volts.

Doctors and radiotherapists at the Christie are eagerly

awaiting a computerised axial tomography X-ray body scanner. This is a further development of the brain scanner designed by EMI. At a cost of £300,000 it could be fifteen years before the Christie has a machine of its own. One is in the process of being installed at the Manchester University Medical School and Christie doctors will shortly be sending a limited number of patients for scanning.

The machine has been described as the greatest advance in diagnostics since the discovery of X-rays. A senior radiotherapist said of it: 'It is revolutionary and a tremendous breakthrough. I hope the inventor, Dr Godfrey Hounsfield, is awarded the Nobel Prize.'

The Christie Hospital and Holt Radium Institute is financed by the National Health Service. Only one third of its money for research is provided by the government. One member of the staff drew my attention to the children's ward which is overflowing with more toys than the children could possibly play with. They have been given by good-hearted folk for emotive reasons, but 'if they really want to help these little ones, they would give the money for research', she said.

Similarly, there is not one water bed – used to relieve pressure points on emaciated patients – at the Christie. The NHS cannot afford them, any more than it can afford to provide the Christie with its own continuation hospital.

My conclusions? That this is a happy hospital with a purposeful, positive approach to cancer – and it is an attitude which rubs off on the patient.

For myself, I am not 'out of the wood' yet, but I view the future with a cautious optimism. But for the staff of the Christie, I would have no future at all.

On the day I returned home from the Christie for a month's rest before starting on a course of drug treatment, I received a card from the Blood Transfusion Service, asking me to give a pint of blood. I am a rare blood group and I have always considered this a worthwhile thing to do.

Cancer made me no longer eligible and I rang to tell them so. A cheerful voice on the other end of the phone said: 'Oh hard luck, dear. Don't worry – when you've had your final check-up and you've been clear for a year, we'll have you back.'

I hope they do.

I SURE HOPE THEY DO!

Headline: The Spiritual Hovercraft that will See Me Through.

One of the nice things about being in hospital – and there are some – is that one's friends send cards, flowers and other gifts which are the tokens of their concern for one's well-being and speedy recovery.

In the course of my work as a journalist I meet a great many people, but it took cancer to make me realise how many of them are my friends. The sheer goodwill and kindliness of our local community overwhelmed me. I broke down and cried. The majority of them added, 'I'll say a prayer for you,' or, 'We'll remember you in our prayers.' People of every denomination have shown to me expressions of their Faith and because of this, I felt as though I went into the Christie on some kind of spiritual hovercraft. This cushion of prayer has sustained me at a time when I have been unable to pray for myself.

Whenever I have been asked 'Are you a religious person?' – something in me revolted. I prefer the word Faith, meaning to have trust. I have faith in the teaching of the New Testament.

In human terms, the words and actions of Jesus are those of a man of sound common sense and sensitivity. He understood his fellow men; he knew their weaknesses and their strengths; their sufferings and privations and their fierce national pride that the impositions of an all-powerful foreign regime could not quell. He understood personal pride, both the satisfaction of a job well done and that denigrating pride which forbids the settling of differences between one human being and another.

To me, the very humanity of Christ is a surety of his divinity. To use his own words out of context, 'If it were not so, I would have told you.' What he promised through his death and resurrection, was a place in his Father's Kingdom. For us, this is the life which comes after our life here on earth.

Why then, if he is a loving God, does he see fit to inflict suffering on the beings created in his own image? I do not think he does.

When one thinks of the machines mankind has made – be they simple timepieces or the intricate machinery that took man to the moon – all of them pale into insignificance when compared to the machine that is the human body. Yet it is the most abused machine of all. We expect it to work when it is tired; we feed it with too much, or too little fuel; we allow it little time for repair or renewal. And still it keeps going, giving us good service we take for granted – until it finally protests.

I am not a doctor and I would not presume to hazard a guess as to the cause of cancer. But I think it is true to say that the average man probably treats his car or his lawnmower with more respect than he has for his own body. Whether some form of abuse is the cause of cancer I do not know. I do not believe it is caused by the Creator. But I do believe that if we will allow him to do so, he can use our suffering for his own purpose.

Cancer. So what then, is the worst that can happen to me? I can die.

When we go out of doors and it is cold, we wear a coat. When we come indoors, we take off that coat. When we die, we discard the body we shall no longer need in the life after death.

But how about the physical act of dying? I cannot imagine

that it is any worse than having a general anaesthetic – a temporary oblivion – then wake up in a much better world where this human form of ours is no longer required.

And what is that new world like? If we can believe what Jesus told us, it is a place of abiding love. Perhaps it is not entirely the love we have known in human terms, but cancer has given me an inkling of the kind of love it might be.

Perhaps it has been just a small lifting of the veil, but it has manifested itself in the close relationships with my husband, my family and my friends. Through the many kindnesses I have received from people, some of whom I do not know awfully well. These relationships and the inate kindness of folk are always there. Yet so often, the pace of life, the mundane, the seemingly important, yet in fact trivial, things, get in the way. Yet adversity can reveal qualities in most human beings which have the nature of the divine. It has taken cancer to make me realise this.

Professor R. W. Luxton, chairman of the Medical Board of the Christie Hospital, put it another way. In a paper he wrote in 1945 he said: 'Man is striving and straining, often blindly towards a better world, a better life, where he will know the cure for cancers of the human body and for the malignant ideas which destroy confidence between men. That he is far from this goal is clear from the present turmoil in the world. May it be that in pioneering a pattern for dealing with physical cancer, there is emerging a pattern for dealing with cancer of the human spirit?'

On the success of the one rests the destiny of individuals.
On the success of the other rests the destiny of mankind.

That was the situation in July 1976. Following the publication of the articles, I sent a copy of them to Mike Marsh, a programme presenter on BBC Radio Blackburn. Would they form the basis of a programme about cancer? Mike was interested. More than interested; later he was to tell me that what followed broke new ground for him and possibly for Radio Blackburn, and that the programme we recorded was one of the most difficult with which he has been concerned.

It was called 'Cancer and Me', but before it was eventually broadcast on 22nd August 1976, John Musgrave, Manager of Radio Blackburn, felt that medical opinion should be sought. In view of the emotive nature of the subject, John was concerned that no listener should be given, however inadvertently, a misleading impression of the causes of cancer, the treatments, the possibilities of cure, and the role and achievements of the Christie Hospital. In short, he wanted a medical 'thumbs up' before authorising the transmission of the programme. Having got both clearance and approval, the programme was broadcast. It was repeated the following evening and was followed by 'Cancer and You' which was a phone-in programme scheduled to last twenty minutes. In fact, this programme ran for forty minutes and when Radio Blackburn closed down, there were still listeners on the line, wanting to ask questions about cancer and to air their views. The studio panel comprised Dr Moya Cole, a consultant of the Christie, Mr Alistair Grant, Deputy Regional Director of the Manchester Regional Committee for Cancer Education, and myself.

The programmes were valuable in that they were another step forward to bringing the subject out into the open, in the hope that they would remove some of the fear surrounding the word cancer.

For several months after the publication of the articles, the *Gazette* office had many requests for copies and so did I. People who suddenly found themselves facing a similar situation remembered them and wanted to read them again. They seemed to find them helpful.

The broadcasts also created a great deal of interest, with many listeners telephoning expressing interest and asking questions. It proved that there was a need which had to be met.

If the first chapter of a book should set the scene for the reader, and if what followed became an eventful and formidable journey, then the articles and broadcasts can be regarded as the pathfinder.

2

Preparation for a Journey

The power of the written word was brought home to me at a very early age by a clout on my ear.

It happened this way.

Our nature-study class at Halton Bank Junior School, Salford, were told to write a composition describing a tree. It didn't matter which species, we could each choose for ourselves. At this point in time, I cannot remember which tree I selected. It must have been some obscure variety. I intended to convey that although it may not be a popular choice, I thought this particular tree was beautiful.

At the age of seven, what I set down in my exercise book, ended with the punch line: 'I think it is a very nice tree, even if you don't.' The teacher took it as a personal affront. Hence the clout. I was carted off to the headmistress, a fearsome old battleaxe, who read me her version of the riot act and I was sentenced to three days of 'solitary' – sitting at a desk in the school hall.

Maybe in the more enlightened seventies a teacher would ask a child what he or she had been trying to express. In 1935, my choice of words was considered cheeky. Come to think of it, I seemed to spend an awful lot of time at that desk in the school hall.

However, the incident gave me a respect for the English language and a delight in the use of words. English and history were my favourite subjects. I was an avid reader of books, comics, newspapers. History books were not just a string of dates, places and events to be memorised, they were stories of people who had lived long ago. In my imagination, I lived in the times about which I read.

On a more contemporary note, I waited with eager anticipation for the day of the week on which the *Girls' Crystal* was published, to read how those story-book heroines of a girls' boarding school had got themselves out of the latest scrape.

I found mathematics a dead bore, which seems ironic for someone who in later years would initiate the raising of a vast sum of money. An insatiable curiosity and a tendency to giggle – usually at the wrong moment – often led to trouble. I remember walking in crocodile down the school corridor and wondering how the flick of a switch on the wall made a bulb light up on the ceiling. No sooner had the thought entered my head, but I must demonstrate to myself the magic of electricity. That desk in the school hall again . . . and nobody explained how this wonder of science came to be.

I was born on St Patrick's Day, 17th March 1928. My mother tells me that my Christian names, Patricia Victoria, were chosen long before I was born. It seems my maternal grandfather had a soft spot for Lady Patricia Ramsay and my Godmother's name is Victoria. The fact that I arrived on St Pat's Day is just coincidental. The Zodiac sign for those born at this time of the year is Pisces, the symbol for which is two fishes, swimming in opposite directions. To my mind they represent the practical and the artistic sides of the Piscean nature – sometimes in conflict and at other times complementary.

I was an extremely healthy little girl, with more energy than most grown-ups knew what to do with. Dark brown hair and eyes and an olive complexion and rosy cheeks, I had an exuberant vitality and an appetite which prompted my Great Aunt Emma to say that she'd rather keep me for a week than a fortnight.

Ours was a happy home. We didn't have much money to spare, but I don't ever remember going short of the things that mattered. I was well loved, well fed and decently clothed. I was a chatterbox and talked my mother's head off with a dogged persistence which frequently brought her to the point of exasperation.

An extrovert, I was not shy. I delighted in the company and conversation of people of all age groups. As an only child, the one thing in my entire life which has ever given me cause for envy is my lack of brothers and sisters. On reflection, I must have been more than a bit of a handful. Maybe my mother and father thought that one like me was enough to last anyone a lifetime. It could have been simply a question of economics. At the same time, I was a sensitive child, easily moved by the misfortunes of others, whether they were characters in the current story book or real people. *Black Beauty* or *Anne of Green Gables* were guaranteed to produce tears. I remember feeling sorry for a little girl in our class whom most of my classmates seemed to shun. I went to sit next to her. After so much time at that desk in the school hall, I knew what loneliness could mean. The friendship was of brief duration. It lasted until I got 'nits' in my hair, much to my mother's consternation. There followed torture sessions with Derbac soap and a fine-tooth comb and strict instructions to sever the association.

If I were asked which one person had the most influence on my early years, I would have no hesitation in saying that it was my maternal grandmother. She died of cancer at the age of fifty-five, when I was seven years old. Gran was the kindest person imaginable and had patience with me when everyone else's had run out. My mother and her three sisters and all the family adored her.

My aunt remembers opening the front door of my grand-mother's house, to find me standing there in print dress and white ankle socks and with my two hands cupped.

'What have you got there?' she had asked.

'I've brought Grandma a handful of sunshine,' I explained.

Gran was a Deaconess at the Salford Central Mission and my earliest memories include Sunday mornings in church with her and going to sleep, leaning against her ample form during the sermons. People never sought her help in vain. She had a maxim: 'If you can't see any good in a person, then don't see any bad.' She was a sweet gentle lady, an excellent cook, a true Christian and a wise, wise woman. I can remember her clearly. Even now, if I am in any doubt about what course of action I should take, I find myself thinking: 'What would Gran have done?'

After passing the scholarship examination, later to be known as the Eleven Plus, I went to Tootal Road School. Here, I established a better rapport with the staff than I had achieved at junior school. Perhaps, being that little bit older. I had learned that discipline was a fact of life one could not ignore. In any case, the War had just begun and the school was evacuated to Lancaster. It brought a closer relationship between children and staff.

As what was known as 'the phoney war' progressed, children and teachers gradually drifted home again. Then came Christmas 1940 and the Manchester and Salford blitz . . . Lancaster homes were again inundated with evacuees. I had a very happy time in Lancaster and was billeted with a delight-ful family with whom I still keep in touch. But all the 'to-ing and fro-ing' made a settled secondary education extremely difficult. By 1942, I was back home in Salford. My diminutive mother was now doing war work, driving a Pool petrol tanker and my father was in the RAF as a groundcrew electrician, servicing Lancaster bombers.

In late 1943 I went to work as a very impressionable junior

in the accounts department of the *Manchester Guardian* and *Evening News* offices in Cross Street, Manchester. One of the highlights of the working day was to be sent with a message or memoranda to that holy of holies, the editorial department on the fourth floor. Here was the heart of one of England's greatest newspapers. Journalists whose names were household words pounded typewriters, telephones and the teleprinters rang incessantly and copy boys formed a human chain between sub-editors and the linotype men two floors below. The quietest corner of Editorial was the room in which Roy Ullyett drew his cartoons for the *Manchester Evening News*. I remember that he kindly gave me a drawing which we raffled to raise funds for our Youth Club.

Also on this floor was the 'inner sanctum' occupied by the editors. Through these doors, famous people from all walks of life could be observed entering or leaving. News of their presence would filter through the building like wildfire but autograph hunting was frowned upon. The *Manchester Guardian*'s fine reputation for accurate journalism was due to the man who was its editor for fifty-seven years, Charles Prestwich Scott. His maxim: 'Fact is sacred, comment is free' was instilled into every journalist he employed.

Maybe the vibrations of the massive printing presses in the basement became too much for the fabric of the old building, for *The Guardian* and *News* are now in Deansgate and the old building in Cross Street no longer exists. Under its new name *The Guardian* the newspaper still upholds the standard of honest reporting set by C. P. Scott. In all humility, I would add to his maxim that if comment is free, it should where possible be kind, for kindness is the food on which each soul thrives and humour is mankind's best tonic.

Eventually, the smell of newsprint got into my nostrils and I began work as a junior reporter on the *Salford City Reporter*. In those days, only senior reporters were allowed 'by-lines'. A cub reporter's copy was printed after much mutilation and

33

revision by the editor (who was akin to God Almighty!) in complete anonymity. Travelling about the city on a bicycle, one was sent to cover church events, meetings of local organisations and also encouraged to produce whatever news one's own initiative could find. The day someone pinched my bicycle from outside the office door was almost catastrophic. In those days, very little of a reporter's work was done via the telephone. Most families didn't have a phone. We went out and met people. It was either shoe leather or a pair of wheels and a face-to-face interview. There is still no substitute for it.

There followed a brief period when I was an ATS driver and it was while travelling in a troop carrier from Woolwich to Folkestone as a passenger that I was involved in a road accident. It meant that optimistic hopes of travel and adventure were quashed; I was invalided out of the service and as souvenirs of this period of my life, I have a metal plate and four screws in my right arm.

Whenever I have been asked 'Where did you meet your husband?' the answer usually produces a smile. We met on the altar steps. It must have been an omen for if ever a marriage was made in heaven, ours was.

My parents had moved from Salford to the village of Bilsborrow, near Garstang, when I was almost twenty-one. The first time my mother and I attended evensong, the Vicar showed us round the church after the service. We were standing in the sanctuary when the local headmaster and his eldest son, Geoffrey, came out of the vestry and we were introduced. Some two and a half years later, on 20th October 1951, Canon Moss finished what he'd started and married Geoff and me.

There followed happy years as a housewife in our cottage in nearby Churchtown village and later when our adopted son and daughter arrived, they were and are a joy to us.

As with any other family, life has not always been a bed of roses. There have been times of worry and stress. Whatever has come along, Geoff and I have faced it together. I have had several sojourns in hospitals. Someone once defined a crashing bore as the person who wants to tell you all about their aches and pains, when all *you* want to do is to tell them about *yours*! For that reason, the reader is not going to get a detailed account of my medical history, except where it has some relevance to this story.

In 1961, we moved to our present home which is one mile north of Garstang Town Centre. When Michael and Helen were both at school, I was offered a part-time job as secretary to the North-West Regional Director of The Missions To Seamen. The Society is the Church of England's oldest industrial mission. My work consisted of administration – receipting donations, answering letters, maintaining a filing system and making appointments for the director, who was out on several afternoons and evenings each week, giving talks or film shows about the work of the Society. The North-West Region comprised over a thousand Anglican churches: the Dioceses of Blackburn and Carlisle and one Archdeaconry each of the Bradford, Manchester and Chester Dioceses. When the director left, it was more than a year before London headquarters appointed his successor.

The Society has a club for seamen on Preston Dock. At this time, the then Bishop of Lancaster was chairman of its committee. Under his guidance, I kept the region 'ticking over'. It was hard work and became far more than a part-time job.

The Right Reverend Anthony Leigh Egerton Hoskyns-Abrahall became my friend and mentor. A man of utmost charm, compassion and sincerity, he has the wisdom of years, the learning of a theologian and the simplicity of the true Christian. Add to this seventeen years of service in the Royal Navy plus a reputation for being an excellent raconteur and you have some idea of his personality. I regard Bishop Tony, as he is affectionately known, with the utmost affection and respect.

Some months after the appointment of a new regional director, I decided that it was time I returned to journalism. Over the years I had, from time to time, contributed to various publications. I no longer wanted a staff reporter's job, with its eighty hours per fortnight discipline. I wanted the freedom of a freelance, able to submit copy where I chose and to have it accepted or rejected on merit and to be able to work as much as domestic obligations and my own inclinations dictated.

Garstang has a population of some 4,000 people. Three sizable towns – Preston, Blackpool and Lancaster – are within easy reach; it has the outer reaches of the Pennines to the east and the Lake District is less than one hour's drive north on the M6 Motorway. It is an ancient country market town surrounded by numerous small villages. It is a good place to live. They say nothing happens in the country and nothing could be further from the truth. One could be out every night of the week in Garstang, for it has many clubs, groups and societies. Wherever there are people, there is always something going on and much of it makes interesting reading for the local community. I report Garstang area news for three newspapers; *Lancashire Evening Post* (Preston), *West Lancashire Gazette* (Blackpool) and for the weekly local edition of the *Lancaster Guardian*. All three papers are owned by United Newspapers, Tudor Street, London.

Garstang also has a thriving Arts Centre housed in a fine building, almost 300 years old, which was formerly a grammar school. Not a grammar school in today's sense of the word, but a place where local children of days gone by were taught the 'three Rs' by tyrannical headmasters who didn't hesitate to use the rod. There are those still living in the locality who can remember being on the receiving end. The building's lofty rafters now provide excellent acoustics for the local choral society and each month a new exhibition of paintings lines the thick stone walls. As one whose hobby is painting, I have been a keen member of the Arts Centre. Endeavouring to create a drawing or painting of reasonable standard is an absorbing pastime. I know that I could never earn a living as an artist and when someone actually asks to buy one of my pictures I am surprised, for painting is something I do purely for pleasure. One is never satisfied with one's own efforts, but it's great fun trying.

For almost ten years I was superintendent of the Sunday School of our Parish Church of St Thomas, Garstang. I enjoy the company of children. Children are *people* – they just haven't lived as long as us adults. Children are like a handful of dolly mixtures, all of them different and all of them sweet. Of course, there's always the odd few little imps who will try to create havoc on the slightest pretext, but they usually found they'd met their match in me. After all, I used to be one, so I was usually one jump ahead of them.

I suppose that mine has always been a practical Faith. I remember when I was about twelve, asking the Vicar of the church I attended if a friend and I could wash the grimy marble memorial tablets lining the walls. We arrived at the church one winter's night, armed with buckets and scrubbing brushes. Having seen us begin, the Vicar left to attend a meeting. Outside, the wind howled through the trees in the churchyard and dark clouds scudded across the sky, periodically obliterating the moon. This was during the war and I cannot now remember what the black-out arrangements were. I do remember that the church was dimly lit and that the silence of its interior was an awesome contrast to the turbulence outside. By the time we had washed the tablets on the north wall, they were as white as the driven snow. So were our faces. The eerie atmosphere proved too much for us. Imagining a ghost behind every pillar, we fled. I wonder if anyone got around to washing the tablets on the south wall? We didn't.

Children have a simplicity, a directness and a clarity of

mind which can stop you in your tracks. Many times, I have been trying to explain some aspect of the Bible as a recipe for living, a pattern for today, when a child has said something which has put the whole question under discussion in a nutshell. I am sure the children taught me every bit as much as I taught them.

Writing infiltrated, as it does in most things. I used pop tunes and wrote hymns to them. Some of my hymns and carols – there's about a dozen – had music written for them by various people. It was because of a hymn to the Van Der Valk theme 'Eye Level' that I first came to know Mike Marsh of Radio Blackburn. I find it difficult to describe myself. I have never really cared for writing in the first person singular. But let's get one thing straight. I am not sanctimonious and I am not a puritan. I enjoy a good social life. I like the occasional drink with my friends and I admit that I smoke more cigarettes than are good for me. I am generally easy going and self-indulgent but there are times when I can 'blow my top' with the best of 'em. I hope I have integrity. I like to think that I have a sense of humour and a sense of fun.

Then in April 1976, along came cancer. It's damned hard to see the funny side of cancer, even supposing it has one. It was to change my life.

The idea of raising money to buy a scanner was not an overnight decision. During successive visits to the Christie outpatients' department, I heard and learned more about this new technology with the unwieldy title. The doctors were now sending a few patients each week to the Stopford Building, where Manchester University Medical School's scanner was housed. The results had been very encouraging and they were extremely enthusiastic about the benefits to patients with certain types of cancer.

Computerised Axial Tomography X-ray Whole Body Scanner . . . the name left the average layman with a glazed expression. Just what was this machine and why was it hailed as the greatest advance in diagnostics since the discovery of X-rays? The technique was a completely new way of seeing what went on inside the human body and with a clarity hitherto unknown, except by invasion of the body, i.e. opening up a patient on an operating table.

Computerised – *via the computer*; Axial – *at an angle, in this case, scans producing pictures*; Tomography – *from the Greek word 'tomos', meaning 'slice'*.

The system was invented by Dr Godfrey Hounsfield, a scientist of the Central Research Laboratories of EMI, the giant concern better known for its vast recording and entertainments industry. Dr Hounsfield first began working on this line of research in 1967 and by 1971 EMI had the world's first brain scanner on the market. It was successful beyond all expectations. The whole body scanner is an extension of this same technology. Both brain and body scanners brought the inventor international recognition and many international honours, including the 1972 MacRobert Award, considered to be the British equivalent of the Nobel Prize for technology.

It is possibly an over-simplification to say that the system is a marriage of computerisation and X-ray photography, for both the technique and the results are vastly different. The images produced by conventional X-rays are shadowgrams that show bone matter clearly, but with the softer tissue organs becoming less clear. CAT uses highly sensitive detectors which measure the strength of fine X-ray beams after they have passed through the patient's body. The computer converts this stream of electronic information into a television-type picture or as a photographic print of a cross section through the patient.

Explaining CAT to audiences, times without number, following the launching of the Appeal, my description would probably have made the technical people cringe. But at least it gave the average person some understanding of how it worked and just how valuable a tool it is.

The scanner treats the human body as if it were a sliced loaf, with the crusts being the top of the head and the soles of the feet. It scans each slice and as information on successive slices is produced, a three dimensional impression is built up of everything within the body. The doctors can ask the computer to enlarge any section of a picture of any slice, should they wish to see it in greater detail.

Seeing the images produced by the CAT scanner you don't have to be a doctor to realise what a miraculous aid to diagnosis it is. Later, I was to nickname it 'Medicine's Magic Eye', a bit of graphic journalese which was to become a catchphrase.

And what about the application of this technology to cancer medicine? The CAT scanner shows cancerous tumours in their size, shape, density and even chemical composition. It improves the accuracy and efficiency of radiotherapy treatment. It's like the difference between buying a suit off the peg and having one tailormade to fit your own requirements. CAT not only offers earlier and more accurate diagnosis for many types of cancer; it replaces certain lengthy and unpleasant tests and can replace exploratory surgery. I know that had I been able to have a CAT scan, there would have been no need for me to have had a laperotomy (open up, take a look) operation at our local hospital, no need for two weeks' hospitalisation with all the discomforts that entails; no need for two weeks' recuperation before being referred to the Christie. The CAT scanner would have produced the information in twenty minutes and I would have been receiving radiotherapy treatment five weeks earlier. Five weeks can be the difference between life or death. In short, more accurate diagnosis, more accurate treatment and the greater the chance of survival. The consultants at the Christie estimate that at least half the 5,000 cancer patients they deal with each year could benefit from CAT.

Well then, why hadn't they got one?

'Because there isn't the money for one,' I was told.

'Won't the National Health provide you with CAT?'

'No, the NHS is broke.'

'In that case, why don't you appeal to the public? I'm sure if people knew that you needed this machine, they'd be only too willing to help. After all, it's in the lap of the Gods – none of us knows if we are going to have cancer in one form or another. I didn't expect to get it, but I've got it!'

'We can't do that. We are not allowed to appeal for public donations.'

'Why ever not?'

'Because of the law. There's a clause in the 1948 Health Act which forbids it.'

So here we had a ludicrous situation. A machine which was a breakthrough of British inventiveness, of similar significance as Roentgen's discovery of X-rays; a National Health Service which either couldn't or wouldn't afford it; the largest cancer treatment hospital in the whole of Europe whose doctors needed it and yet were unable to let the public know of that need. There is an old saying 'the law is an ass'. It was never more of an ass than in this instance.

'How much do you need?'

I was told that it would require half a million pounds. The basic scanner was £300,000 an additional computer for radiotherapy planning would be another £50,000 and, as the Christie was already chock-a-block, a new building would have to be found at an estimated cost of £150,000. Total, half a million.

One of the consultants said to me: 'One day, these scanners will be standard equipment in every general hospital, but it won't be in our lifetime.'

Half a million pounds is a lot of money by any standards. But how do you equate money with lives saved? You don't.

My fees for the *Gazette* articles and the Radio Blackburn broadcast had been sent to the Christie. It was my way of saying 'thank you' for the excellent care and attention I had received. When my consultant had first read the articles, he had said: 'I wish I could write like that.'

'You can mend bodies. Your work extends life. Which is more important?' and with a grin, I'd added: 'Sooner or later they'll be lighting the fire with those pieces or wrapping fish and chips up in them. That cuts any journalist down to size.'

However, the *Gazette* management had told me they intended to enter the articles for the Journalists of the Year Awards. The results would be known in January 1977.

I now had a greater appreciation of the hospital's need for CAT and slowly, an idea was germinating in my mind. If by some chance, the articles did win an award, I'd give the cash prize to the Christie, letting it be known that it was towards the purchase of a scanner.

Meanwhile, I would continue to do what I could to eliminate fear.

For a few months, life resumed some measure of normality. I started working again. I was on drug therapy. Every couple of weeks, Geoff and I drove from Garstang to the Christie. Each time we passed the high wire fencing before the Wythenshawe exit of the M63, I felt as though cancer was closing in on me. I was no longer a person, but a patient. Even now, that stretch of motorway has the same effect. I know it is purely psychological but I cannot drive along there without that same feeling. Coming back along the M63, knowing that the medical report had been 'so far, so good' gave a feeling of blessed relief. For another two weeks, I could forget hospital.

It wasn't to last for long.

In October, my mother's sister died of cancer after twelve months' illness. In November, my mother had two thirds of her tummy removed, plus a tumour, fortunately intact. During her stay in hospital, my father lived with us. We had mother home for only three days when Dad fell down our staircase and broke a rib. December 1976 and life assumed a degree of unreality. Family events began to seem like a series of cartoon drawings in a horror comic. The thought of Christmas, with all the extra work it entails for a housewife, filled me with dismay. I couldn't eat, and I was tired, oh, so tired.

The 23rd December and my parents' Golden Wedding Day. I recollect that we gave them a small party and I remember a superb arrangement of yellow flowers on a small table in our sitting room.

My next recollection is of the Christie Hospital on New Year's Eve. What happened to Christmas 1976? I have no memory of it.

When one has a dark olive complexion it is difficult to tell how much is jaundice and how much is natural colouring, for I look suntanned all the year round. Suspected gall bladder trouble turned out to be another tumour.

On the credit side, ovarian-type tumours respond well to radiotherapy, but they do have an insidious habit of throwing out small satellites and it is difficult to know where they are until they cause trouble. The latest one was obstructing the tiny passage between the liver and the bile duct. To be insensible on an operating table is not the ideal way of getting blotto on New Year's Eve. More surgery was to make my torso look even more like a page out of the AA handbook with Spaghetti Junction thrown in for good measure. That was the least of my worries. At almost forty-nine I had no desire to wear a bikini.

The surgeon inserted a drain tube to by-pass the bile duct. New Year's Day came and went and so did ten more days before I was considered strong enough to take more radiotherapy. Meanwhile, the bile drained into a bag, through rubber tubing protruding from my diaphragm. Food was

43

utterly abhorrent. I survived, first on a drip feed and then on oral liquids. The smell of the food container arriving in the ward was nauseous to me.

I am an impatient patient and any ward sister's *bête noire*. Even though desperately ill, enforced inactivity drives me up the wall. I couldn't raise any interest in any form of occupational therapy; I couldn't even be bothered to read. At night, I couldn't sleep and spent many hours in the darkened day room, smoking one cigarette after another and drinking cups of tea supplied by sympathetic nurses.

Early January is just about the drabbest and most depressing time of the year. Lying in my bed, I looked out of my window as fog came down, along with the darkness, as daylight drew to a close. Visitors would have a hard time of it, getting to the hospital tonight. The thought of Geoff driving fifty miles down the motorway to spend half an hour with me worried me. On the mobile telephone, I rang him at the office and told him not to come. 'It's not worth it in these conditions. I wouldn't know a moment's peace if I thought you were trying to get here in thick fog.'

That night, there were less than the usual number of visitors in the ward. I resigned myself to being one of the patients without anyone. Then a familiar face appeared. It was the friend of my childhood, Beryl Acton. We had been friends since we were six years old and we were both at Halton Bank School.

'Have you driven here in this fog?' I asked her.

'No, I came by bus. It's too risky by car tonight. I'm glad Geoff hasn't taken a chance on it.'

'So am I.'

We chatted and, as old friends will, reminisced about things that had happened over the years. Beryl had brought all kinds of dainty titbits in an attempt to get me to eat, but I just couldn't face them. As we talked, I asked if she was cold.

'Heavens, no. It's like a hot house in this ward!'

I didn't seem to be able to find the energy to sit up. I began to shiver and shake.

'You need attention. I'm going to find a nurse.'

The staff nurse came, covered me with extra blankets and gave me a dose of brandy and rang for a doctor.

'Beryl, promise you won't tell Geoff. There's no point in worrying him when he can't get here. The hospital will call him if they think it's necessary,' I pleaded, between chattering teeth.

I was given a wide spectrum antibiotic; blood samples were taken and analysed and after the bug was identified, I was put on the appropriate antibiotic. Thus, pneumonia was averted.

Later, Beryl was to tell me that she went home and cried, thinking it was the last time she would see me and that a friendship of over forty years was about to end. True to her promise, she did not telephone Geoff. By the time we talked on the telephone the next morning, things were under control. My poor husband had quite enough to worry about. And the worst was yet to come.

My consultant had prescribed eight daily treatments of radiotherapy. After the second of these, he came to see me.

He looked troubled.

'Pat, come into the office. I want to talk to you.'

I got out of bed, put on dressing gown and slippers and tottered down the corridor. In the office, I sat facing him across the desk.

He told me that things didn't look too good for me. He was sorry to have to give me such bad news, but in fact, he had to tell me that I was dying.

Dying? *Dying?*

Every now and then, life deals us a blow which sends us reeling. This one pole-axed me. Knowing that you have cancer, you also know that there is always a possibility that it might kill you. But to have it spelled out for you, not as a possibility, but as *certainty* . . .

I asked him how long I'd got and he said that he couldn't say exactly. It varied between one patient and another. I looked at his face, and his expression was one of kindness and concern, but with an element of defeat.

I thought, 'What a hell of a job this is for him.'

'It must take some doing, to have to break this sort of news to a patient?'

'It's not easy. It is something one never gets used to. Of course, one couldn't tell every patient in your circumstances but I know you'd rather have the truth, Pat, than be fobbed off with plausible explanations.'

My first thought was for Geoff, the man I loved and whom I'd seen age ten years in recent months. I didn't want to leave him. How could I tell him *this*?

'You'll have to tell my husband. I can't do it. I just can't.'

It is said that when one is confronted with death, all of one's past life passes before one's eyes. It's true. Back in bed and with the screens drawn, I put my head underneath the sheets and cried. In those few square feet of privacy, memories flitted across the mirror of my mind. I thought of the day we met. Courtship, marriage, bringing up the children. All the happy times we'd shared; the laughter, the comradeship, the arguments, the jokes. The times when Helen, scoring some lively debate around our dining table as though it were a tennis match, had interjected with 'fifteen-love, fifteen-all' . . . so much happiness.

The same dining table, complete with a small hole made when Geoff and a much younger Michael had got over-enthusiastic with a drill when making model aircraft. I remembered their crestfallen expressions and the scolding I'd given the pair of them. All the little things, the treasured memories of our family life. So much happiness . . . oh, dear God, was it all going to end? And now our children were young adults. What would they do with their lives? I thought

46

with unutterable sorrow about the grandchildren I would never have the opportunity of knowing and loving. I thought of my parents, both of them far from well and worried sick about me, doing their best to help keep my house going. One chick and all their eggs in one basket. This would break their hearts. They must never know, until the truth became impossible to conceal.

Vera the nursing auxiliary came and found me. She put her arms round me and let me cry it out. Eventually, I slept through sheer exhaustion. At visiting time, Geoff, my mother and a friend arrived and I tried to behave as normally as possible. I should have got an 'Oscar'. In the few minutes we had alone together, I told Geoff that the doctor wanted to see him. Our eyes met. We never have been any good at keeping secrets from each other. The relief of being able to share the burden was beyond words. Heartbroken, we decided that knowledge was strictly for the two of us. We'd face it together.

The morning of the seventh treatment and the worst day of all. I was now three stones below my normal weight. I looked like a scarecrow, my hair was a mess and my morale at rock-bottom.

'I can't go on. I can't fight any more. I just want to be left alone!'

My consultant tried to rally my resources. Only the dregs were left. 'Pat, this isn't a bit like you. You've only one more treatment after today. We're trying to buy you some extra time. Come on, now. Where's that fighting spirit of yours?'

Fighting spirit? How did I know where it was? I wouldn't have cared if I'd died there and then.

The eighth treatment and the bag was removed. The end of the drain tube was clamped off with a heavy lead clamp known as a gate clip and which could have anchored the *Titanic*. The tube was wound in Catherine-wheel fashion and taped to my chest. Was the tumour inactivated? Would the bile duct function normally? And if so, for how long?

A couple of days later, I was allowed home. It was the 22nd January 1977.

On the 1st February my son was twenty-one. I managed to stay up for part of the family gathering we had that evening but eventually had to go to bed and leave them to it.

When others were there, Geoff and I put up a front. When we were alone, we clung to each other, sharing a grief beyond words.

February 1977 and my battle with myself . . .

So you're going to die . . . so what? Everybody does it. It's the one appointment we all have to keep sooner or later. You don't want to keep it any more than anyone else, but it doesn't frighten you, does it?

No, the thought of dying doesn't frighten me.

It's the thought of leaving your family that fills you with dread, isn't it?

Yes. Oh yes! I love them all so much.

It may be sooner than you wanted it to happen but there's nothing you can do about it.

I know. You don't have to tell me.

Well then, what are you going to do? Sit there on your backside, worrying yourself sick and making the whole family miserable in the process? Is that what you want?

No.

You can sit and mope or you can get on and make the most of every day as it comes along. Make the most of the time you've got eft! You're not dead yet, girl. So get on with it – and LIVE! What have you done with your life so far?

Nothing of any great importance.

No. You're just Mrs Average. You've enjoyed the good things and weathered the bad patches. So do other people. You aren't the only one who has troubles. Stop feeling sorry for yourself and do something positive.

48

You are quite right, conscience, but do what?

Well, what about that scanner you've heard so much about?

Yes, but the *Gazette* articles didn't win. There's no cash prize to give the Christie.

What about it? You've used your talents before and given the money to the Christie. What are you going to do with them now? Put them in a box and throw away the key?

It'll take a lot of time. I'd rather spend it with Geoff and my family.

THINK, woman, think . . . what have you to offer? You value family life, don't you?

You know I do.

There will be plenty of other men, women and children who will have cancer. They love their families just as much as you love yours. How about them?

Yes, how about them . . . but half a million pounds . . .

Half a million pounds, mocked my conscience. *You haven't got half a million pounds and as you don't fill in the coupons, there's not much chance of your winning the football pools is there?*

What CAN I do?

Your job is the communications media. Start communicating. See what other people will do to help you. This isn't the sort of thing you can do alone. But you could get it started.

Get the thing started . . .

Yes. The ocean is made up of small drops. If you can get an Appeal off the ground, maybe there'll be enough folk who will see fit to carry it on when you disappear from the scene.

Could it be done?

How are you ever going to know unless you try?

What had I to offer? Previous experience of charity work. I knew how a charity should be organised. If I started a fund for this scanner, I would need as much representation as I could muster. The area served by the Christie extended from Barrow and Kendal in the north, to Crewe and Wrexham in the south. If I could get one person, or a group of people in

49

each area interested . . . But *would* people be interested?

All of life is an experience, most of which we file away in our mental library, never knowing when we are going to have to take some of the books down off the shelf and use them. My mind went back across the years to my childhood and to Christmas 1940. The phoney war had come to an end. Until now, the German word *Blitzkrieg* had tripped uneasily from British tongues, but the reality shortened it to 'blitz'.

For night after night during what should have been the season of peace on earth and goodwill towards men, enemy planes circled the skies above Manchester and Salford. The first portent of coming disaster was usually the wailing of the air-raid siren. The ominous sound of those rising and falling notes were echoed in the pit of one's stomach. Next would come the drone of a single plane and then the blackout would be pierced with the light of parachute flares. Instead of the Star of Bethlehem, searchlight beams swung about the heavens, as the German bombers came within their orbit and ack-ack gunners tried to blast them out of the sky before they could drop their deadly cargo on our cities. Incendiary bombs and high explosives rained down on us, with the enemy concentrating much of his attention on the industrial complex of Trafford Park. The glow of burning homes and factories seemed like the interior of hell itself. Most terrifying of all were the land mines, floating down remorselessly and silently on parachutes – until they hit the ground with a force which made it seem as though the very earth itself would disintegrate. Fire fighters strove desperately to bring thousands of infernos under control and rescue teams worked with an energy they never knew they possessed, digging out their fellow citizens trapped under tons of rubble. Ambulances, picking a way through streets whose road surfaces were like colanders, avoided bricks and debris which only minutes before might have been a neat row of houses or a factory floor. Any of them could have been the target of the next stick of bombs. The dead were taken to the morgue and the injured and dying to hospitals and makeshift reception centres. There was no safety anywhere. As the daylight hours came, the German planes headed back to their homeland – to refuel and reload bomb bays in preparation for the next act of destruction the following night.

And what had been the reaction of Mancunians and Salfordians? In the daytime, we took stock of the situation in which we found ourselves. Shops with hurriedly nailed up boards where the windows used to be, displayed notices which read: 'business as usual'. On the remaining walls of devastated buildings, the graffiti of 1940 read: 'Down – but not out!' or, 'You can bomb us but you won't beat us Mr Hitler!' and a whole variety of other defiant phrases. It was a time when neighbour helped neighbour. He would dig you out of the rubble which had been your home or help you to patch up the windows, shattered by bomb blasts. She would find something for you or your kids to wear if your home or your wardrobe had literally gone up in smoke. We lent or we borrowed our neighbour's butter, sugar or tea ration and bedded down on his living-room floor if ours no longer existed. And incredibly, some of it even had its funny side, for it is a trait of British character that in times of stress or crisis, our sense of humour surfaces.

Dire necessity and a common adversary brought a togetherness, a community spirit, hitherto unknown. It was a fight for survival and, in spite of the humour which kept up our spirits, beneath it all was a cold, bitter fury and a determination to hit back in whatever way we could.

As a child of twelve, I had lived through all this. I had watched my parents trapping incendiary bombs – which rolled down our avenue like milk bottles – with sand bags or buckets of sand. (Get back in that shelter and don't you dare come out again until we tell you!) In our shelter, the seven-year-old girl from next door and I listened to the whistle and crunch of bombs and to the din of the battle raging outside. We clung to each other when a house a few yards along the road got a direct hit, the shelter rocked and our candle went out.

The spirit of 1940 . . . was it still there? I thought it was. People don't change all that much. Only this time, the adversary wasn't Hitler, it was cancer. I found myself filled with a very similar fury against this devil of a disease which splits up more families than the divorce courts. The shock of being told I was dying had flung me to the floor, but the count hadn't yet got to ten. I could pick myself up and go another round. I wasn't beaten yet. I'd give the insidious old ogre a run for his money before I threw in the towel. But I needed every bit of help I could get. Inevitably it would be an emotive appeal – a terminal cancer patient appealing for a machine to help other cancer patients. I could see my colleagues of the Press having a field day with that one. As a journalist I knew it was a good story. The only trouble was, the story was ME. Yet I knew that an Appeal of this kind would need a great deal of publicity if such a vast sum of money was to be found. It couldn't be done unless it was brought to the attention of the public. And what better way could I think of, than to use my own plight to illustrate the urgency of the need?

Did I want to be at the centre of this kind of publicity?

No. I didn't. I'd rather be behind the headlines than make them. Essentially, Geoff and I are very private people. This would be the last thing we would choose if it were for ourselves. And another thing, organising a scheme of this magnitude was going to take up my limited strength and my limited time. Time . . . my most precious possession. Time . . . the commodity in short supply. Whatever time I had left, I wanted to spend as much of it as I possibly could with Geoff and the family. But I knew that I was in a position to do what needed to be done. Whenever there is a genuine need, there is generally someone who comes along to fill it. The more I thought about it, the more I became convinced that the person was me. And bit by bit, a determination to grapple with cancer was overcoming reluctance.

Geoff and I discussed it at length and tried to think of all the implications. Eventually, he said that if I was convinced that this was what I must do, then I should do it. He is the first to admit that at this time he was sceptical, but he thought that having a positive objective, something to aim for, would be good for me in that it would take my mind off my own problems.

Geoff is the most loyal person I know. Once having agreed that I should attempt what seemed an impossible task, I knew that he would back me to the hilt. And as always when faced with a crisis or dilemma, I sought the counsel of Bishop Tony. On 1st March, we had a long discussion at his home, Pedders Wood, and he gave me his blessing. Thus encouraged by two men I loved and respected, the decision was made. And if I was to live with that wretched conscience of mine, I had no choice at all. Whether people responded, would be a matter for individuals, groups and organisations to decide. They had freedom of choice.

I wrote to Lord Barnetson, chairman of United Newspapers, asking for his help and I rang my friend Mike Marsh on BBC Radio Blackburn.

'Mike, who do we know on "Look North"?'

3

The 'Scanner Trail' Begins

BBC Television's 'Look North' film crew took one look at the large airy day room set aside for them by the Christie administration and decided that it looked more like a five star hotel. Instead, they settled for the office next door, which by comparison, had the proportions of an Oxo cube. Into this location, they crammed floodlights, a camera and tripod, sound equipment and enough electric cable to encircle the globe. The room already contained a desk, a steel filing cabinet and a large crate of surgical dressings. It was hot and claustrophobic. There was the camera man, the sound engineer, Liz Donnelly who was to interview Dr Ian Todd, Consultant Radiotherapist, and myself.

I had been told to arrive at the Christie for 2 p.m. After a brief run through, filming would begin at 2.30 and the whole thing would be over by 3.30 p.m. when I was due in the radiotherapy department for yet more treatment. Geoff left us all to it and went in search of a cup of tea.

As we were waiting for the crew to sort out their equipment, Dr Todd told me that half a million pounds wasn't going to be enough. The target was going to have to be three-quarters of a million pounds.

'Three quarters! For heaven's sake, why?'

'Because even if we got enough money for the scanner and the building, the North-West Regional Health Authority couldn't afford to run it.'

'Oh no.' I stared at him in dismay.

There was a silence. A depressing silence. Half a million was a daunting target. Now we needed half as much again. But it was no good getting 'up tight' about it. All we could do was to make a start. See how things went, see what reaction there would be. Maybe eventually we could persuade the government to make some contribution. 'Oh well, if it has to be three-quarters of a million, three quarters it is.' Both figures were mind-boggling, anyway.

Liz interviewed me to get the patient's angle and concluded by saying: 'Pat is not only a patient of the Christie Hospital, she also raises money for cancer research. The need at the Christie at the moment is . . .' and she went on to talk with Dr Todd about the CAT scanner.

The BBC's policy is not to handle direct appeals for money other than on the Sunday night spot designated for this purpose. 'Look North' could only do the programme from the point of view of its news value. Bless 'em, they bent the rules almost to breaking point. If people couldn't put two and two together and make four, it was a 'poor do'.

Finally, the cameraman needed some outdoor shots for the opening sequence, over which an introductory commentary would be recorded in the studio. It showed me walking into the hospital grounds, pausing to look at the sign 'Christie Hospital and Holt Radium Institute' and then entering the main reception door. I did this four times before the cameraman was satisfied, by which time I was exhausted. It was ten minutes to five before I got to the radiotherapy department.

The item was filmed on Wednesday, 9th March and was screened on Tuesday, 15th March. I watched it, crippled with pain. Apparently cancer patients are prone to shingles and I was one of the unlucky ones. From my hip, down to my right foot – I felt as though I had been punched and scalded. I was in for a month of hell that was worse than anything the Christie had thrown at me. I wouldn't wish shingles on my worst enemy.

Meanwhile, the initial response was encouraging. Even before the item was screened, the *Gazette*'s 'Seasider's Diary' column had carried a piece about the filming session at the Christie. It brought an immediate reaction from readers. Letters expressing their good wishes, their affection, their moral support and donations amounting to some £200 poured into the *Gazette* office. These were forwarded to me. I went to my bank, the Garstang branch of the National Westminster and asked to see the manager, Mr Geoffrey Ball. I explained to him what had happened and what I hoped to achieve. What did he advise? An account was opened in the name of The Pat Seed Appeal Fund. I called at the Post Office and bought my-self a supply of stamps and went home to answer the letters, which included National Westminster receipts for donations.

Then after the 'Look North' item, came a response from viewers. Within a fortnight the Fund balance was over £2,000, the Christie administration office also having received donations for the scanner. These were initially paid into their Endowment account, earmarked for the scanner.

In February, Mr Bert Brierley, a Garstang businessman who knew of my intentions had given me £1,100. Bert is the most generous of men. He had built up his firm, Briercrete, from scratch, through hard work and business acumen. He owned a fourteen-bedroomed house, set in its own grounds and materially he was a success. Most things which could be bought with money were his for the asking. But his wife Phyllis died of cancer and this contribution was Bert's memorial to her. Over the coming months Bert was to help the Fund many times. His initial donation had also been paid into the Christie account.

I conferred with the Hospital Secretary, Mr David Critchley. I wanted Appeal Fund money kept entirely separate from any other hospital funds. It was a personal appeal with a specific objective and I thought it would be better 'all under one roof' at Garstang National Westminster.

I quote from a letter I received from Mr Critchley: 'With effect from 13th April, 1977 all donations received in this office and identifiable as being for the Pat Seed Appeal will be recorded, but then banked in the Withington Branch of the National Westminster Bank, Ltd. for credit to the Account No. 04024982 at Garstang. All donors will, however, receive a letter of thanks from me, plus information about the C.A.T. Scanner. As at the closing of the Pat Seed Appeal Fund in the Endowments Account on 12th April, the balance in hand was: £2,720.80p plus £1,100 from Mr. Brierley. When your Trustee arrangements have been finalised, this amount can be transferred to the credit of the Garstang account.'

David was later to tell me that at this time, he was sceptical about the whole thing. He thought raising three quarters of a million was an impossible task. He also said that Geoff Ball had said to him: 'If you think that, then you don't know Pat Seed.' I am not sure just what Geoff meant by that and perhaps it's as well not to ask.

But David was not alone in his thinking. I sensed an attitude of 'OK let her try, but she'll never do it.' And who could blame people? I was not even sure myself. All I knew was that every pound that came in was one pound nearer the objective. Whether that scanner would ever be installed at the Christie, was anyone's guess at this stage. All we could do was to plod on, travelling hopefully.

At this point, neither I nor anyone else knew that what we were seeing was the start of what I was later to refer to as The North-West Miracle. It was like casting a pebble into a pond. The ripples were to spread in an ever-widening circle. I could not have foreseen that I was in for the busiest, most hard working, most eventful period of my life. Nor could I have foreseen that it would be a rewarding and enriching experience.

Keith Daniels of Radio Blackburn came to interview me. This was two weeks after the 'Look North' item and the Fund stood at about the two thousand mark. During our recorded conversation I explained that there was no hope of the NHS providing the Christie with CAT for up to ten or fifteen years. If cancer taught one anything at all, it was to face life as it was, not as one would like it to be. The only way the hospital could hope to get this machine – and lives saved as a result – was by our own efforts. The broadcast brought the comment from a gentleman in Darwen that the machine for which I was trying to raise the money, only cost as much as a missile slung under the wing of a military aircraft.

A lady in Grange-over-Sands had been listening to the broadcast as she sat at home sewing. She wrote to say that she had intended to leave the Christie a legacy. Instead, she thought the money could be put to good use now. Letters also arrived from many parts of east Lancashire. I went to the Post Office and bought more stamps.

As soon as I felt up to the journey into Blackpool, I got a friend to drive me to the *Gazette* office. I had asked to see Sir Harold Grime, Editor-in-Chief. I acquainted him with the progress of the Appeal and mentioned that I had written to Lord Barnetson. Paternal, kindly and courteous, the patriarch of the *Gazette* gave me every encouragement. Having lost both his wife and his mother with cancer, he had reason enough to know what a destructive scourge it was. He telephoned Lord Barnetson's secretary and added his own addendum to my letter. He advised me to write one article on the lines of the series of four which I had written the previous year, but with the emphasis on the need for the scanner. This would be sent to the London office for syndication throughout United Newspapers, most of whose publications were in the north-west. This was just the kind of help I needed.

Before I left the *Gazette* office, I went into Editorial to see my friends, many of whom had sent me cards and flowers during my stay in the Christie. In the coming months, they were to back me to the hilt, both by reporting the progress of the Appeal and by their own personal efforts.

In Garstang, local people rallied to me and to my project. At St Thomas's Junior School, the children had been making things to raise money towards the school's Lent Charity which had not then been named. One or two of the children asked the staff if they could give money to Mrs Seed's Appeal. The idea swept like a forest fire through the school, to such an extent, that the headmaster arranged a morning market in the school hall, to which parents were invited. This was the first organised function I attended in aid of the Fund. It raised nearly £200 by the spontaneous efforts of children under eleven years of age. Trying to express my gratitude to them was very difficult. Many of those little ones were children I had taught in Sunday School. Love your neighbour? Here they were doing just that.

Garstang housewife Mrs Nora Whittingham was one of the first people in the town to do something to help. After seeing the 'Look North' film, she thought she'd have a raffle and asked local business people if they would donate prizes. Their generosity was such that Nora's house began to look like Aladdin's cave and she began to get cold feet. She came to see me.

I gave her a letter to say that she was acting on behalf of me and the Appeal, which restored her confidence. Eventually, we had an auction which raised several hundred pounds.

In the coming months, I was to find the two words 'thank you' increasingly inadequate. How does one thank people who have not only given money, but who have given so much of their time, talents and energy, and who have given of themselves?

At our Garstang Soroptimist Club, fellow members asked,

'How can we help you?' Some gave me stamps, to help cope with the increasing amount of mail. As a club, they decided to organise a mammoth raffle and enlisted the help of every other Soroptimist Club in the North-West and South Lancashire Divisional Unions. The raffle was drawn at our joint conference at the Imperial Hotel, Blackpool on 1st May and together with a tombola it realised more than £1,600.

As the weeks went by, other Garstang organisations offered help and eventually there was not a club, group or organisation which hadn't held some kind of fund-raising function.

At the end of March, a nice thing happened on the home front. The phone rang one night and it was my cousin Clifford on the line. Cliff was the nearest I ever got to having a brother. He had emigrated to Australia twenty-seven years previously and I had not seen him for twelve years. He was in the UK for a six-weeks' visit, spending his time looking up the family and old friends. He came to see us on 30th March and stayed overnight. He had a whistle-stop tour planned down to the last detail. We spent most of the time reminiscing and looking at old photographs. I said that as I probably wouldn't be around the next time he came to England, I ought to merit more than one visit. We arranged that he should spend a weekend with us in April, which he did. It was a happy time.

Perhaps it is as well that we cannot see into the future. Some months after his return to Australia, Clifford died of a heart attack. He was forty-seven and had looked as healthy as one could wish.

When one faces death, material possessions become unimportant. Only people matter. True happiness lies in the friendship, the affection, the comradeship between one human being and another. Yet so often, possessions possess people.

It seems so odd that one so vibrantly alive as Clifford should be dead and a lame duck like me is still in the land of the living.

At the beginning of April, my thirteen-year-old dog, Sherry, died. It was cancer. Dear God, does even the dog have to have cancer?

Following the initial response to the Appeal, I asked Mr Critchley if we could have a notice on the wall in the out-patients' department of the hospital, to let people know of the Fund's existence. OPD is one of the busiest parts of the hospital. Patients – more often than not, accompanied by relatives – arrive for medical or treatment appointments throughout each day starting from nine in the morning until about four thirty in the afternoon. In the course of a week, some hundreds of people pass through the department. These were people who had more reason than most to be interested in such an Appeal.

David shook his head.

'Sorry, can't be done.'

'It can't be done? Why?'

'Because of the law,' he replied. 'We're not allowed to advertise.'

The law is an ass? It was the understatement of the year.

This was 1977. The Health Act had become law in 1948, when my National Insurance stamp was 7s. 1d. Twenty-nine years later, the law was unchanged, even though circumstances were so vastly different and contributions to the NHS had soared.

'Look, David, I'm not trying to rob the place, I'm trying to help. Surely the powers that be realise that? Just how inflexible can they be?'

'I know you're trying to help, but there's nothing we can do about this one. We can't change the law and this hospital has to abide by the rules laid down by government.'

'I appreciate that as an administrator your hands are tied. I'm sorry, but I'm not prepared to let the matter rest there. My hands aren't tied. Maybe we can't change the law, but I'm going to have a damn good attempt to get some relaxation of the rules on this one. It's like living in cloud cuckoo land!'

I had no wish to become involved with politics, to do battle with bureaucracy or take on government departments. All I was trying to do was to raise money for a scanner and that was a monumental task in itself. But, damn it all, if the government couldn't find the cash there was no reason why it should obstruct whatever progress could be made by voluntary means.

After some ferreting around, I got hold of a copy of the Act and also a photostat of a 'confidential' memorandum, issued in 1948, just before the Act became law. Before the Welfare State, hospitals had relied heavily on voluntary bodies. I quote:

'The financial position of hospitals in the National Health Service is *free from doubt*. All ordinary expenditure is met from the Exchequer, including captail expenditure; and hospitals are therefore in no way dependent on voluntary financial help for their normal needs.'

A further paragraph of the memorandum states:

'The direct or indirect participation of Boards or Committees in appealing for or collecting funds for their hospitals – however careful the terms in which any such approaches may be made – will inevitably create the false impression that hospitals in the Service are still dependent on voluntary financial help to keep them going. Accordingly, Boards and Committees should be careful that they do not either directly or indirectly invite contributions. The following are examples of practices which should cease, if they have not already done so:

a) Advertisements in the Press or elsewhere (existing posters should be removed).
b) Requests to individual subscribers by letter or otherwise.
c) Placing of collecting boxes in railway stations, public

houses etc. (any boxes still out should be brought in at once).

d) Requests to patients for donations; contributory schemes conducted by the hospitals themselves.

e) Radio appeals, flag days, bazaars, fetes etc.'

This was the pie in the sky of a free health service – in theory, first class. Unfortunately, it hadn't worked out that way. Almost thirty years later, the Health Service was anything but free and this clause had never been repealed. The law was way behind the times. With the exception of children and old age pensioners, 'Mr and Mrs Britain' now paid for a percentage of prescriptions, spectacles, dentures, etc., in addition to the weekly or monthly deduction from wages or salaries. In spite of vast sums of money contributed in this way the Health Service was anything but perfect.

One frequently heard about the shortage of nursing staff, nurses and junior doctors being underpaid, the brain drain to overseas countries which offered better remuneration and better research facilities. On the other hand, one heard of hospitals looking for something to buy with what was left of their annual allocation of money – it *had* to be spent, otherwise the allocation might be cut in the next financial year.

The public had heard it all before. It was nothing new. No doubt members of the medical profession and the staff of every sector of every hospital have their own theories as to what could be done to improve the efficiency and the economy of the Health Service. They could probably make lists, or write dissertations on the subject as long as from here to Kingdom Come.

I wasn't trying to set the world to rights, or even the NHS. But this business of 'no advertising in the Christie' bugged me. I was blowed if I was going to let the matter rest there. That weekend, I telephoned Mr Walter Clegg, Conservative Member of Parliament for North Fylde. When he came to see me a few days later, we discussed the subject at some length. I gave him copies of the relevant documents and he promised to see what could be done.

At the next meeting of the Standing Committee for North-West Regional Affairs in the House of Commons, on 27th April 1977, Mr Clegg raised the question with Mr Roland Moyle, the Minister of Health. Mr Moyle replied that he would look into the matter. In a written reply to Mr Clegg, dated 19th May, he wrote:

'Mrs. Seed had indeed set herself a daunting task in seeking to raise £750,000 and I should say first of all that I applaud her efforts and feel strongly that the NHS should welcome gifts which they can usefully employ for the benefit of patients and staff. Such a tangible expression of community interest and goodwill does a great deal to lift local hospital morale. It is for the individual health authorities to decide whether or not to accept literature or appeals posters for display in their hospitals. However, in making such decisions, health authorities will have regard to the nature of the appeal and the need to ensure that in no way patients feel under any obligation to contribute, particularly at a time when they may be under some stress. It would be inappropriate and inopportune to put patients in such a position.

'I see no reason why health authorities and district management teams should not encourage local fund-raising activities by individuals, voluntary organisations and community groups and help to ensure that the fund-raising efforts are related to the real needs of local hospitals. Nor do I see any objection to them providing modest facilities to these groups, such as the occasional loan of health service premises, to help them promote their work.'

Mr Moyle also wrote that the paragraph which states that authorities should not invite financial help from the general public for hospital services 'either directly or indirectly' is perhaps a little too restrictive.

His reply was certainly more attuned to the circumstances of the seventies and it put the onus fairly and squarely on the Manchester Area Health Authority.

At the end of July, an informal meeting was arranged between four members of the Area Health Authority committee, Mr Critchley, Dr David Greene, Principal Physicist of the Christie and myself. The members were interested to hear about the Appeal and the numerous events which were taking place. I remember it being mentioned that the hospital did have other needs as well as a need for a CAT scanner. I remember that I replied to the effect that if that was the case, why not list them all, under the heading, 'How you can help *us* to help *you*'. Maybe that was asking for too much without reference to the full committee, but on a show of hands, they gave permission for a discreet notice of the Appeal to be placed in Outpatients.

I had no thought of having scored a victory. My one thought was that at long last, common sense had prevailed. We hadn't changed the law, nor had we broken it. We had bent the rules sufficiently to fit the circumstances of the time. The notice helped to spread news of the Appeal and because of it, the financial contribution has been immeasureable.

In any case, law or no law, this is a free country. I agree entirely with the Minister of Health that patients should in no way be harassed or feel under any obligation. But if they see fit to help, try stopping them – in several wards in the hospital, blissfully unaware of the impediments of the law, patients were running raffles, making and selling items of handicrafts and so on – and they paid the money into the Fund.

Mr Clegg, as well as representing the people of North Fylde in Westminster, is also a solicitor and when I asked him if he would handle the legal side of the Appeal, he very kindly agreed to do so.

He pointed out to me that in the event of my death there

would be difficulties with regard to withdrawal of monies from the Fund. No one else had authority to do so and some provision should be made for this. My original thoughts were that four of the consultants of the hospital should be trustees of the Fund. But by the end of May and after talks with Mr Ball, Mr Critchley and the doctors, it was decided that a Central Committee of the Fund should be formed. Mr Clegg favoured the latter suggestion, because he thought it would take some of the responsibility from my shoulders.

Until such a committee could be formed, he recommended that a Declaration of Trust be signed by myself and one other person whom I should nominate, to state that we held monies in the National Westminster Bank, Garstang, for the Christie Hospital. Legally, this would cover the position until such time as a Trust Deed could be drawn up and the Fund registered as a charity. So, as an interim measure, Dr Ian Todd and I signed a Declaration of Trust. A copy of this was lodged, under seal, at the Garstang Nat-West. It was dated 16th June 1977.

Meanwhile, the money was beginning to earn some interest and Mr Ball recommended that a Petty Cash account be opened. Discussing this, I said that I was sick and fed up with charities where a large percentage of money donated disappeared in administration costs before the residue was used for what it was intended. Mr Ball agreed wholeheartedly, but he pointed out that there was a limit to how long I could subsidise the Appeal out of my own resources. The Fund had to be self-supportive, and should meet all legitimate expenses such as postage, stationery, telephone calls and travelling.

It made sense. Yet I was determined that if people gave a pound to *this* Fund, that's what would go to the Fund. Every letter to which I replied, meant at least a 7p stamp and few people thought to include a stamped addressed envelope. I became frugal, cheeseparing and downright miserly, questioning every $\frac{1}{2}$p we spent, and I have never regretted this attitude.

4

The Path Widens

The Appeal was beginning to be known in the circulation areas of the newspapers for which I worked and by those who had heard the broadcasts on Radio Blackburn, but there were still vast areas of the north-west whose population was still unaware of its existence. I particularly needed to get it known in the Manchester area. How to set about it?

The City of Manchester . . . that historical centre of northern industry, commerce and trade whose bustling streets were among my earliest memories. Piccadilly, Deansgate, Market Street . . . brightly lit shop windows displaying wares of every conceivable size and kind. My earliest memory of Manchester is of being taken to Lewis's store at the age of three, to see Father Christmas. I remember wondering why his whiskers weren't real and how on earth an old gentleman of such vast proportions would ever get down our chimney on Christmas Eve. And were the fairies who helped him *really* as old as that?

As I grew up, the cinemas on Oxford Street came into my orbit. I remember being taken to see a Shirley Temple film and coming home feeling envious and inadequate. She was The Perfect Child. In contrast to those bouncing golden curls and her ability to charm grown-ups into instant submission, my straight brown bob (cut short in case of 'nits') was the bane of my life and my daily misdemeanours a source of shame. Later still, there were shows at the Manchester Palace and the Opera House on Quay Street was another venue of delight, especially when it was the D'Oyly Carte season. Sullivan's lilting melodies, and, even more to my taste, W. S. Gilbert's robustly dexterous words. Oh, to have such mastery of language, such ability to captivate and enthral the listener with the product of one's pen. As a teenager I was transported into a wonderful world of make believe – romantic, improbable, satirical but always magical. To this young aspiring writer, W. S. Gilbert's lyrics were the pinnacle of perfection.

Only later came the realisation that he probably burned as much midnight oil as any other writer as he searched for some obscure rhyme or acceptable scan. Behind the excellence of his craft and those tongue-twisting stanzas, there was much hard work. For writing *is* hard work. Talent, inspiration, creativity all are necessary, but the ingredients for which there are no substitutes are application and staying power. In the final analysis, any writer is on his or her own; there is always the blank sheet of paper. No one can fill it for you. And to my mind, there is no rapport between brain and pen unless the heart acts as mediator.

Mikado, Gondoliers, Pirates of Penzance, etc., can still take me back across the years to a seat in the gods at the Manchester Opera House.

Memories too, of my teenage years at the *Manchester Guardian* and *Evening News* building on Cross Street. Thirty-odd years later, I didn't know anyone on the editorial staff. It would have to be an 'ad'. I made enquiries and found that a four-inch two-column spread would cost about £100. Should I risk it? Would it do any good? The *Manchester Evening News* had a massive circulation and I had to make a start somewhere.

And anyway, what was money? There are no pockets in a shroud.

The advertisement appeared as a single-column small type-set notice that wouldn't have attracted the attention of a fly crawling across the page. I rang our local agent who had handled the 'ad' for me and asked for a repeat insertion, but in the format I had ordered. The next thing, the phone rang and I had my first conversation with Duncan Measor, editor of 'Mr Manchester's Diary'. During my time at the *News*, Duncan had been fighting the war as a naval officer. That was why our paths hadn't crossed. Now, he'd seen the proof of my advert.

'You're NUJ, aren't you?' (National Union of Journalists.)

'Yes.'

'Well, what are you bothering with "ads" for? Why didn't you send us some copy?'

'Because I don't know anyone on the *News* these days.'

'Then it's time we got acquainted. Now tell me all about it. Tell me what you're trying to do.'

I told him. Duncan listened sympathically. Like the experienced journalist he is, he knew that he'd got a good story. (Only don't mention the fact that I m dying, will you? My parents don't know about that bit.) He then spoke to the consultants at the Christie and sent photographer John Holland to Garstang. At the beginning of April, the Diary Column carried the story, together with two pictures; one of me taken about the time I worked at the *News* and the other showing me holding cheques sent for the Appeal and which did not NOT show the long skirt I was wearing to hide the shingles. That was the beginning.

A couple of weeks or so later, I met Duncan in the foyer of the *Manchester Evening News* offices on Deansgate and he took me across the road to the Manchester Press Club for a drink and a chat. He says that he remembers that day, grey and overcast and with a steady drizzle draping a dripping mantle over the city. It provided a setting which was about right for what he describes as one of the greatest gaffes of his life.

'There you were, thin and frail, hardly able to stand. I grabbed your arm and plunged you amid four lanes of traffic with words I'd used many times before when piloting others across Deansgate: "Come on – die with me!" Later, I shuddered at the enormity of its callousness. There hadn't been such a boner since a journalist joined our paper twenty years ago and on his second day in the office had enquired of a colleague, "Who's that ugly fat woman over there?" and back had come the paralysing answer, "My wife!" Fortunately, all you did was laugh.'

Months later, Duncan was to tell me that his diary column was going to Seed!

As the Appeal progressed and more and more support was fothcoming from *News* readers, the stories came into his office thick and fast. 'Suddenly,' said Duncan, 'the world was full of people wanting to give their widow's mites, their pocket money or their pensions. What you had planted was growing in a way that would have made old Jack give up planting his beans!'

Come to think of it, I never did receive an account for that advert.

Bert Brierley rang me in early April. How would I like to meet Red Rum? *Would I?* Of course I would! Bert owned three racehorses which were under the supervision of Don McCain at his Southport stables. He was driving over to cast his eye over them and to discuss prospective races. He said that he rather thought there might be a donation to the Fund. I asked Bert if it would be in order to let the Press know and he said that it would.

Shortly after we arrived at the stables, Don had to leave to attend a race meeting, so it was his wife Beryl who introduced me to the triple Grand National winner. Here was the horse who had become a legend in his own lifetime; the creature who had made world-wide racing history. What a magnificent animal he is. His chestnut coat gleamed. Grace, beauty, strength, courage and intelligence in one aristocratic equine frame. He's a personality. He's a poser as well. He knows what cameras are all about. As Mrs McCain presented me with a cheque on behalf of the stables and as photographers recorded it, Rummy's ears pricked up and he could have been any film star meeting the Press. As soon as the photographers had got what they wanted, it was almost as though he switched off his smile. Then his stable lad mounted him and they headed for the yard gate, en route for his morning exercise. When they returned, we were in Beryl's kitchen and as Bert discussed business with her, I stood by the window from which I could see Rummy's stall.

Stable boys were playing with him, winding a leg bandage round his muzzle. As playful as any puppy, Rummy was enjoying the game as much as any family pet. He's the darling of the stables and a firm favourite in more ways than one.

The first charity night I attended on behalf of the Fund was at the Chequered Flag Hotel, Garstang. It was to be the fore-runner of many similar events in hotels up and down the region and it was a riotous evening. Yorkshire comedian Charlie Williams topped the bill. He was hilarious and during his act heckled a chap who was trying to eat chicken in the basket with remarks such as: 'Haven't you finished that *yet*?' and, 'You've not left much for the dog, have you?' The audience loved it, the diner probably got indigestion and the Fund benefited by about £375.

The three papers for which I reported had each given their readers news of my attempts to raise money for the scanner and in early June, United Newspapers syndicated my article. Each editor was free to use it as he chose. The *Wigan Observer* printed it as it stood and their Woman's Page editor, Val Belshaw, whom I had known when she worked on the *Post* in Preston, telephoned. 'Anything I can do to help, just ask. Keep it going, love!' Val had a call from reader Barbara Steane, also a cancer patient and a couple of weeks later, Val featured Barbara in her column. On the *Post*, Muireall Kelt used the article in 'Womanpost' and pledged her support. The editor of the *Burnley Express* gave the article to journalist Winnie Bowes. Winnie decided to use it from the local angle. As a member of the Soroptimist Club of Burnley, she knew that a fellow member, Mrs Julé Hayward, was also a cancer patient. She called on Julé and showed her my piece and asked for her opinion.

'Right. If she can come out into the open, then so can I.' – and Winnie told readers Julé's story. Following this, Julé wrote to me to ask how she could help me. 'Let's get this scanner installed!' I telephoned her and asked her if she would like to start a Burnley branch of the Fund and to this she readily agreed in spite of her considerable disability. She became an indefatigable worker. During the course of our initial conversation, I said: 'You know, all it really needs is a million people who would each give 75p and that would be it. But life's not like that, is it? It's going to depend on the people who see fit to do something about it. Many folks just won't want to know.' Julé remembered this long after I'd forgotten it. Later, her brilliant idea was to bear bounteous fruit.

Gazette reader Margaret Parkinson wrote to me and agreed to represent the Fund in Blackpool. I had known Margaret when she lived in Garstang and the Appeal renewed our friendship.

In the Borough of South Ribble, a young girl, Suzanne, decided to hold a garden party, having read about the Appeal in the *Post*. Her mother, Mrs Helen Dickinson, wrote to me and in July, she and her husband, Robert, formed a South Ribble branch of the Fund.

Following publicity in the *Lancaster Guardian*, Ted and Sheila Warburton of Hornby called to see to offer their help.

It was growing . . . things were really starting to move. The mail now came with elastic bands round the letters and our postman told me I had my own pigeon hole at the sorting office. Our longwinded address was abbreviated to 'Pat Seed, Garstang, Lancashire', and the phone rang incessantly with enquiries or offers of help. The *Evening Gazette*'s Women's Circle arranged an afternoon meeting at the Imperial Hotel, Blackpool. This was attended by two of the consultants of the Christie and myself.

Between us, we gave as much information as we could, about the cancer and about CAT. Later, many of the ladies organised their own fund-raising efforts and sent their cheques to the Fund.

In Hornby, Ted and Sheila had arranged a Flea Market in the village hall to which they had invited Geoff and me. As we approached the tiny hamlet, we were astounded at the number of cars parked on the main street.

'My stars! What's going on? Just look at all these people!'

'There's probably some other affair going on in the village,' said Geoff.

But there wasn't and the local constabulary were having a hard time of it, for trying to find space for all the cars was like trying to squeeze a quart into a pint jug. Inside the hall, there seemed to be every conceivable item under the sun for sale and Ted had asked a bank-manager friend from Kendal to act as auctioneer for the more valuable items. The hall heaved with people, packed like sardines in a tin and all prepared to be generous. Suddenly, the responsibility of it all overwhelmed me. What had I started? It was frightening to have motivated so many people. I knew that the cause for which I was working was honest, right and, hopefully would eventually benefit cancer patients of the future. Who was I? Just plain Pat Seed, a middle-aged housewife and mother. Right now, Pat Seed was nervous. Any set speech I had in mind went to the four winds. There's only one way, in my experience, to cope at times like this and that is just to be oneself. If one tries to be anything else, one is likely to come a cropper. I explained as simply and sincerely as I could, what the objectives of the Appeal were and that success depended on the goodwill of people from all walks of life. Speaking to audiences at meetings, gatherings or functions since that night at Hornby, I have never used set notes or speeches. I can only speak from my heart spontaneously to individuals, whether there are 30, 300 or 3,000 people present. I either get the point across or I don't. I can only be myself. That has to suffice.

A great deal of hard work by a great many people lay behind the success of that night at Hornby. Ted and Sheila and their helpers were all worn out when it was over, but they had a great sense of achievement. The Flea Market had sent the Scanner Fund soaring by another £1,700 – all this from a tiny village, the main street of which is hardly more than about 300 yards long.

At Appley Bridge, Barbara Steane and her friends from the local pub, the Hesketh Arms, held a Gala Day. There were numerous stalls and side shows, tug of war teams, pony rides, etc., and a local DJ played disco music. A lovely sunny Sunday ensured success. It was here that I met Audrey Brindle and Megan Abraham, both of whom were patients of the Christie. They both offered to help. Megan had already had a CAT scan at the Manchester University Medical School and knew the worth of the machine for which we were trying to raise money. She founded the Shevington branch of the Appeal and Audrey formed the Wigan Central branch.

And so the Appeal was off the ground. By mid-July 1977 I had done just about everything I could think of and the amount raised in four months was £30,000. It was a fine start, but oh dear, that three quarters of a million seemed as far away as the planet Mars. How long was it going to take? Even supposing I lived that long, I could be grey-haired and in a bathchair by the time there was sufficient money. *Come on, God, it's your turn. What do I do next?*

But before I tell you what did happen next, let's take a look at the home front.

There are three very natural reactions to being told that you are dying – shock, helplessness and fear. It is truly amazing just how much human beings can take. Even when confronted with a shock of such enormity, such finality, the mind, little by little, adjusts. Geoff and I *had* to come to terms with the facts whether we liked it or not. What alternative had we? Eventually, we devised a philosophy for coping with the situation in which we found ourselves. But more about that later. Helplessness was to a large extent overcome because I was trying to use the experience in a constructive way.

Fear? That is a continuing battle and is a many sided thing. There is the fear of dying, the fear of pain, the fear of being a burden to those one loves. These fears are not exclusive to cancer patients. Anyone who is seriously ill, whatever the complaint, has these fears to a greater or lesser degree. But for so many people, the word 'cancer' has with it a nightmare quality not associated with other – and sometimes far worse – complaints. For some, cancer has a stigma as though it is something of which we should be ashamed. I have heard of people who have hidden themselves away, being too embarrassed to admit that what was wrong with them was a form of cancer. I don't know why this should be so. There are people with multiple sclerosis, diabetes, heart trouble, arthritis who, with little hope of a cure, are not ashamed to admit they are so disabled. Like other complaints, cancer is a malfunction of the body. It is a word, but it is not necessarily a sentence. It is a collective noun, the overall term for malignancy of body cells. I remember asking a consultant just how many types of cancer there are, and she replied, 'You could say there as many as there are cells in the human body.' No one yet knows what triggers off cancer, causing body cells to go awry. If scientists knew that, they'd be a whole lot nearer to finding an overall solution. As it is, some forms of cancer are curable and while research progresses in many directions in an effort to find that common denominator, much still needs to be done in cancer education.

And who better to help bring the subject out into the open than those who have it? I resolved to do just this, as much as I could, when meeting people who were helping my Fund. The Appeal could be used for this dual purpose, for fear was an adversary against which I myself was fighting. By fighting my battle in public, maybe I could be of some encouragement to others.

During my trials and tribulations since April 1976 my family and my friends had rallied round me, giving me all kinds of practical help and moral support. I was fully aware that in some respects, the situation was far harder for Geoff than it was for me. How agonising it must be to stand by and watch someone you love suffer, not only in a physical sense – and that's bad enough – but to watch them try to face up to the fact that death itself may be just around the corner. I know that if our roles were reversed, I would want to shoulder the burden for him, have cancer for him, rather than watch him have it. I guess this is how Geoff feels about me. That is not possible but, bless him, he's done the next best thing. He's been the rock upon which I've leaned and the one person to whom I could tell every waking thought and his has been the shoulder to cry upon when morale broke down. The words of the marriage service come to mind: 'To love and to cherish in sickness and in health until death us do part.' I am loved. I am cherished. Therefore I am blessed. In spite of everything, what more could any woman ask for?

It's funny how the passing of the years reverses the roles of parents and children. When we are small, parents are protective. As the years progress, we gain independence along with adulthood and as our parents grow older still, we become protective towards them. It is hard now to imagine that my frail little mother had driven an ambulance during the blitz and later, a heavy Pool petrol tanker. The shock of learning that their only daughter was dying could prove too much for my parents, now in their late seventies. As far as they were concerned, the medical verdict was 'wait and see'.

But there were just a few people to whom I could talk freely and in these early days, they provided the safety valve I needed. One was my friend Tess Pickford, a former staff reporter on the *Lancaster Guardian* whom I have known for some twelve years. As a freelance, I have worked in close co-operation with Tess on the Garstang edition of the weekly paper. Many a Wednesday night would find the pair of us racking our brains, trying to find a good lead story in time for the noon-Thursday deadline. Some weeks, when the news flowed and when there had been plenty of local events, the problem didn't arise. At other times, we would be scraping the barrel, doing a mental tour of the district, seeking new ideas or new angles on earlier stories. Eventually, one or the other of us would come up with something which, even if the sub-editors took a jaundiced view of it, did make a front-page lead. We know most people in the district, all of whom came under our probing and, for the most part, kindly scrutiny. Work like ours is never boring and to my mind, the essential requisite of any journalist is not an ability to string words together – although it helps! – but to have a genuine interest in, and love of, people. Tess shared this opinion. She is one of those gregarious characters who thrive on company. Combine this with a vivid imagination and the unexpected becomes the norm. Life with Tess could never be dull. It could be highly improbable, but *never* dull. I remember a Christmas when our branch of the NUJ decided to hold a fancy dress party at a Lancaster Hotel. Tess had decided to go as 'The Guardian Angel' and had codged up a white nightie and halo. The wings were a headache. We spent a whole night, cutting out leaf-shaped pieces of gold contact paper and sticking them on to a wire frame. Getting her into the car with them was a devil of a job. We overcame the problem by chucking the wings in the boot until we got to the hotel. I wore a red dress, covered in tinsel and Christmas decorations and went as the Spirit of Christmas. After several hours of hilarious festivity, we came out of the hotel in the small hours of the morning, much to the astonishment of a passing motorist who couldn't believe his eyes and almost drove over a roundabout.

In her spare time, Tess ran one of the local Cub Scout packs of which Michael had been a member. She arranged an annual Father and Son camp. It was a weekend packed with imaginative, adventurous activities. Dads and lads had a whale of a time, but the former came home worn out and aching from head to foot, having used muscles they'd forgotten they possessed. Tess's thirst for adventure meant that for most of the year, she saved up madly for her annual holiday, which was always spent in some far-flung foreign clime. Who else could come back from their holiday, saying that they'd met Moses on Mount Sinai? Yet it was true. Holidaying at a Red Sea resort, she had climbed Sinai and had happened to meet a young man called Moses. Her holiday anecdotes usually made a good feature for the paper on her return. During the times when illness prevented me from working, Tess dropped in to see me two or three times a week, bring some small gift of flowers or sweets and a fund of amusing stories, none of which either of us would dare to print. Then in April 1977 she dropped her bombshell. Her predilection for foreign parts had prompted her to apply for Voluntary Service Overseas candidature. September 1977 would see her setting course for the Solomon Islands where she was to run a school for journalists and write for the local paper and radio station. I knew that I would miss her very much. There was also the depressing thought that I might never see her again. However, our friendship would continue by letter and there was nothing more certain than that hers would make interesting reading.

The other good friend is both a guardian *and* a ministering angel, although that is the last way she would describe herself. I refer to Marie, my district nurse. In the spring of 1975 I wrote a series of articles 'Women At Work', featuring local ladies who, as well as looking after their homes and families, held responsible jobs or professions. Marie was one of them. Her home is on the other side of the road from our house and until that time we had just had a nodding acquaintance as neighbours. This particular evening I had gone across to her home, armed with notebook and pencil, expecting the interview to take half an hour or so. Two hilarious hours later, I was still there. Anecdote after anecdote poured out of this pint-size Florence Nightingale and after nearly every one, I had to say, 'But I couldn't possibly print that!' I remember her telling me about a time when she had to give evidence in an accident case, to which she had been a witness. Never having been in court before, she was in such a state of nerves that she addressed the chairman of the bench – who happened to be Lord Lyle – as Sir Tate. 'Well, I knew it had something to do with sugar!' It seems that after some dialogue which would bring the house down if it were the script of a TV comedy show, she was asked to leave the court as her evidence was of no use to either the prosecution or the defence. The Press were in paroxysms of mirth and I have no doubt that Lord Lyle had a smile on his face. Tears of laughter streamed down my face and as I hadn't got a handkerchief with me, I asked Marie for a tissue. 'Here – have one on the National Health,' she said, passing me a square the size of a card table. I had great difficulty in finding something for that article that *was* printable.

The result was headlined: **Why Marie's a real tonic.**

'If your idea of a district nurse is a formidable woman who weighs around 17 stones and has half a dozen chins – forget it and meet Mrs Marie Calvert. She is four feet ten and a half inches small and seven stones seven pounds of cheerfulness. If I were unfortunate enough to be ill and confined to bed, there is no one I'd rather have visit me than Sister Calvert, who is a member of Garstang's District Nursing Team. She would do me more good than a bottle of medicine. As well as being a highly efficient member of the nursing profession, with eighteen years of experience behind her, Marie has one of those engaging personalities. She would have you smiling, even if you were at death's door.

'In private life, she is Mrs Eddie Calvert and the mother of seven year old Nicola and two year old Timothy. Her working day begins at about eight-thirty when she takes Nicola to school and leaves Timothy with Grandma. She is attached to one of Garstang's busy medical practices and works in co-operation with four doctors. She visits an average 15–20 patients a day and earlier discharges from hospitals have meant a heavier case load in recent years. Two or three evenings a week she is on call until 10 p.m. Marie says that a lot of people mistakenly think that District Nurses are a quack branch of the profession and "wouldn't you like to be a proper nurse in a hospital?" is a familiar question. Yet district nurses are hospital trained state registered nurses and state certified midwives. They have usually had at least two years as ward sisters before going on the districts.

'Marie Calvert has seen the joy of new born life and witnessed the sorrow of life's closing moments. She brings to her work a warm friendly personality and a sympathetic understanding of the problems sick people and their families have to face.

'Yet Marie says that she herself is accident prone and cars are her *bête noire*. "I have lost count of the number of minor mishaps I have had and if ever I run out of petrol, it is usually in the middle of the A6 when I am about to turn right." A policeman told her that she doesn't park her car – she abandons it!

'She recalls being taken on the back of a tractor down a rough farm track to a cottage to attend a maternity case. The tractor easily negotiated the deep muddy ruts, but the driver lost his passenger and her equipment. Marie found herself sitting in the middle of the track and the farmer had arrived at the cottage before he realised that his passenger was missing.

'If she ever chose to write her memoirs, they would have best seller potential. Meanwhile, life is too busy for Marie Calvert, housewife, mother and a popular highly respected member of one of the most honourable professions a woman could choose.'

Little did I realise, when I wrote that article, how eternally grateful I was to be for Marie's ministrations. Twelve months later, she not only attended me professionally, she was the friend who helped me during the initial shock of cancer. Her sound common sense, spiced with her ready sense of humour, has been a Godsend ever since. There is nothing funny about cancer, yet times without number we have been helpless with laughter over some aspect of my plight. When I came home from the Christie in January 1977 I couldn't have a bath unless Marie came to help me for I had not the strength to cope by myself. And that wretched drain tube with its heavy clamp, we nicknamed the Titanic, for I felt sure that if by some mischance it went down the plug-hole, I would follow it. It was a most uncomfortable piece of apparatus. I couldn't wear a bra. Not that it mattered. I was so thin I'd nothing much to put in a bra, anyway.

In fact, being thin was something of a novelty. One night I

took my wedding dress out of its box and tried it on. I hadn't been able to get into it for over twenty years and I decided to give a Geoff a fashion parade. Later, seeing his expression, I realised it was an insensitive thing to have done and I could have kicked myself. Fat or thin, I could never again be the slim young girl who had worn it to walk down the aisle as his bride. He would rather see me my normal size-sixteen-struggling-not-to-be-a-size-eighteen and WELL, than have me a size twelve again with one foot in the grave.

As my strength began to return with the help of drugs, I was able to bath myself. Marie and I had a routine. After my early morning dip, I would hop back into bed and ring her number, allowing the bell to ring twice. This was the signal that her first case of the day was ready for her. Many times, she has walked into the bedroom, only to find me answering another phone call. Pulling a face at me instead of a polite 'good morning' she has fixed the Titanic and left me still in conversation with someone about the Appeal.

'It's a damn good job this isn't television!' would be her comment the next time she saw me.

If she thinks I am overdoing things, she is a miniature martinet. She is quite capable of pinning me to the mattress, drawing the bedroom curtains and taking the phone off the hook with the words: 'And don't you dare move from there until I come back or I'll send for Dr M—! Where's that diary of yours? You're not going anywhere tonight!' And as she lives just across the road and can see any movements in or out of our drive, I have little choice in the matter.

I remember an occasion in February 1977 when I was thinking about launching the Appeal. Marie, Tess and my mother and I were drinking cups of tea in our sitting room. I was worried about coming out into the open and the kind of publicity it would entail.

'I suppose, when one thinks about it, it's going to be a prostitution of my own difficulties.'

My mother, for whom the word 'prostitution' has only one connotation, looked horrified. Aghast, she had said: 'Oh Pat, you wouldn't do a thing like that, would you?' We laughed until we cried. Bewildered, mother had asked, 'What are you three laughing at? I didn't say anything funny.' – which only made us laugh all the more.

Since my dog Sherry had died, I had been longing for her successor. At one period when the children were younger we had so many animals about the place, I threatened to put up a notice at the gate, which said 'Zoo'. I also promised myself that one day, I would write a book entitled 'Animals Who Have Owned Me'. For starters, there had been two pet owls and a Mynah bird with a disconcerting vocabulary, so I had no shortage of material or characters.

Now, with Sherry gone, we hadn't any animals at all and the place just didn't seem like home without at least one pet.

'Why don't you get a dog from the RSPCA?' suggested Helen, who was home on a visit.

'You know what would happen, don't you? I'd either come back with their entire stock or be so upset I'd cry for a week!'

I fancied a King Charles spaniel. One day in May, Geoff rang from his office to tell me that a colleague had just bought one and there were two puppies left in the litter. Would I like one? I didn't need asking twice and that evening, on the way to see them, he said: 'Now think on – this time, it's to be ONE pup, not two.' The last time we had gone to choose a dog, Mike had liked one of the litter and Helen another and we'd ended up bringing them both home with us. Amber had died three years ago.

'Do you think you are up to coping with a puppy? Will it be too much for you?'

I was adamant that I could manage and the following morning, Bonnie Boy came into my life. In repose, he looked like a soft toy exhibit that had just won a first prize at a handicraft exhibition. Mike said that all he needed was a zip fastener along his tummy and he'd make a good pyjama case. The trouble was, repose didn't last very long. Most of the time, he was a squirming, wriggling bundle of copper and white hair, with flailing paws, needle sharp teeth and a tail like a piece of chewed string. He had an insatiable curiosity and gave every visitor a boisterous welcome. They usually went home with either laddered tights or tattered shoe laces, but as he was such an engaging little fellow, most visitors readily forgave him. He quickly cottoned on to certain facts: the kitchen means a full tummy; the garden and NOT the best Axminster is his loo; his new basket, which he systematically frayed round the edges, is his own special domain, and the perfect place to hide his treasures, including a squeaky effigy of Harold Hare and anything else he thinks is his. He found that father's armchair is a jolly sight more comfortable than the floor, only surpassed by the comfort of my bed. One of the first things he learned was that he could twist me round his chubby little paws.

Geoff and Mike seem to have ended up with so many odd socks that you'd think the house was populated by a crowd of Long John Silvers.

'That dog gets away with murder!' my husband complains, although he spoils Bonnie as much as the rest of us.

Bonnie Boy is now two and he's still more like the court jester, not yet having acquired the dignity of his royal breed. His appetite is reminiscent of an animated vacuum cleaner. There are times when I have to remind him that his famous namesake ended up having his head chopped off and he'd better watch it! His mature coat is beautiful – long and silky and he has a thick ruff. That 'piece of chewed string' is now an elegant plume and at just the right height to swipe everything off the coffee table. Consider all this, his appealing, expressive spaniel eyes and his sunny nature and it's small wonder that I adore him. Mike, who would never admit to loving him, *will* refer to him as 'Bozo' and says that he's a hooligan.

13th April, the date of a profound experience.

Some weeks earlier, during our conversations at Pedders Wood, the Bishop had recommended that I should have the benefit of the Church's Sacrament of the Anointing of the Sick. He said that he would prepare me for it and that he would conduct the service in his private chapel.

'You will either be cured, or you will be given the strength to face whatever the future holds for you.'

I remarked that it would be so easy to be proud of what I was trying to do. I recognised a need for humility.

'Pride is a very human failing. Put yourself in God's hands as his humble servant. Allow him to use you as he will, for with him, all things are possible. Remember that you are merely a tool, an instrument. You have recognised your need for humility. Accept it – and forget it.'

So, on the evening of Wednesday, 13th April, Geoff and I drove to Pedders Wood accompanied by our Vicar who was to assist with the service. The only other person present was the Bishop's wife, Margaret.

I make no attempt to describe the service. There are some things which are beyond description. It had been truly a sacrament, leaving Geoff and me with a greater insight into that familiar phrase, 'the peace of God which passes all understanding'. The words of the twenty-third psalm took on a new significance. 'Though I walk through the valley of the shadow of death, I will fear no evil. Thy rod and thy staff comfort me . . . Thou anointest my head with oil; my cup runneth over . . .' Suddenly, it was all right. The worry was taken away from me and in its place I had peace and a new philosophy. I had been given a job to do. I knew, from that moment on, that I would be given the strength to do it. What is more, I knew that I would not be doing it alone.

Cured? I didn't know. It no longer seemed to matter. All I knew was that I was in God's hands and there was no further need to worry. Worry . . . what is this thing called worry? The human race spends an awful lot of time doing it. What if this happens . . . what if that . . . and half the time the things we worry about don't happen. If they do, that's when we're stuck with them and that's when we have to try to sort them out. Worry is a negative waste of nervous energy. It is a quite different thing to 'concern' which is a positive emotion with a practical application. We may regret some of the things which happened yesterday, but no amount of worrying will alter them. No one appreciates that more than me. As Omar Khayyam put it: 'The moving finger writes; and having writ moves on: nor all thy piety nor wit shall lure it back to cancel half a line, nor all thy tears wash out a word of it.' That old boy knew what he was talking about. As for the future, there's not much we can do about that either, for the simple reason, it's not yet here. By that, I do not mean that we should not be prudent or that we should make no provision for the future. To opt out in that sense would indicate a lack of responsibility and even the ultimate in pessimism.

But so often it is all too easy to fall into the trap of imagining all kinds of hypothetical situations and to worry ourselves to a frazzle about them when the chances are that most of those situations will never arise.

Therefore, all we are left with is TODAY. Whether you've been told that you are dying of cancer or that you can expect to live for another sixty years, no human being can live more than one day at a time. Whatever the set of circumstances with which we are faced, *this day* is the only day we can deal with them effectively.

The New Testament puts it as a simple Truth: 'Why worry about tomorrow when today has sufficient cares of its own.' Like many other simple truths, its very simplicity causes it to be overlooked, underestimated, ignored. And yet its simplicity is its wisdom and its wisdom its strength. It is a basic ingredient of happiness.

Does it come as a surprise to know that in spite of having been told that I am dying, I am happy? That's no heroic statement. It's true. Here, I will try to analyse my thoughts. As I have already explained, death itself doesn't frighten me. I regard it merely as a shedding of the form I will no longer require in the life to follow. And if I am wrong, and there isn't a life after our life here on earth, then it won't matter anyway. If I am afraid of dying, which, like birth, is a perfectly natural process, then I am also afraid of living, for fear of dying. And if I am afraid of living, I am not going to live my life to the full; I am not going to enjoy the good things, for fear they may end or be taken away from me. Another thought is that life doesn't owe us a living. There is more satisfaction in giving and in what we are able to contribute than in what we can grab. Each human being enters this life with nothing other than the talents with which he or she is born. Admittedly, circumstances, fate, destiny – call it what you will – plays a part in shaping the paths each of us will tread upon this earth. Some of us will have more of this world's goods than others, but really, whatever we possess is only on loan to us, for in the final analysis all each of us really owns is that which lies within ourselves.

On what we do with those talents, will depend our own fulfilment, our relationships with other people and what contribution we can make to society.

So I have cancer. I am surrounded by a kind and loving family all of whom are concerned for me and all of them as supportive as they can be. Yet they cannot have cancer for me. *That is something I have to do by myself.* And sitting wondering whether today, tomorrow or the day after tomorrow might be my last, isn't going to change a thing. It will only prevent me from making the most of TODAY. A TV interviewer asked me. 'What's it like, living with death?' I replied, 'I wouldn't know. You tell me. I live with life.' Therefore, I am NOT dying of cancer. I am LIVING with it. Dying only takes a second, the space between one breath and the next, which is conspicuous by its absence. Am I going to worry about that? No. There's a heck of a lot of living to be done before that final breath and when it does come, I hope I can meet it with dignity and tranquility. Meanwhile, 'One Day At A Time' is my recipe for life. And when you pause to think about it, can any one of us do more? There is nothing of the 'Holy Joe' about me. But I do have a very sincere Faith which goes beyond Sunday lip service to as practical an interpretation as I can muster. Sometimes I succeed better than at other times. Far from making me question it, my experiences have strengthened Faith and have given me a contentment of spirit, an inner peace. Some may find that incomprehensible, but it is this which helps me to overcome fear. Shock has abated; helplessness has been replaced by a sense of purpose. Fear, like Faith, has to be worked at, constantly.

To say that I am *never* afraid, *never* depressed, would be to try to bamboozle the reader into thinking that I am either superhuman or half witted. I am neither of these. Along with a capacity for jumping into things with both feet (and often finding myself involved up to the neck!), I think I have some measure of adaptability and a resilience which has stood me in good stead. I am a natural optimist but when bouts of depression descend on me, as they do from time to time, I try to find some absorbing thing to occupy my mind until depression has passed. Sometimes it works. Sometimes it doesn't. I am an ordinary woman, putting the best she can offer into each day as it comes along – ONE DAY AT A TIME.

Some time ago, I came across the following lines. I have no idea who wrote them or whether they are subject to copyright, but I think the writer would not mind me quoting them.

This is the beginning of a new day.
God has given me this day to use as I will.
I can waste it, or use it for good.
What I do today is important, for I am
Exchanging a day of my life for it.
When tomorrow comes, this day will be gone forever,
Leaving in its place, something that I have traded for it.
I want it to be gain, not loss;
Good, not evil;
Success, not failure, in order that I shall not regret
The price I paid for it.

As a writer, I wish I'd thought of those wise words. But
I can learn from them.

How many days are left to me, I do not know.
But do you, dear reader, do YOU?
The time to be happy, is NOW.

5

Some Exhausting Progress

Shortly after the initial 'Look North' interview a young man from Manchester's commercial radio station, Piccadilly Radio, had recorded a conversation with me. He was now working as a freelance for the BBC's Radio Four programme, 'Today'.

In mid-July, just when I was wondering what to do next, the phone rang. It was Mike Hopwood asking if he could drive over to record an item for this early morning feature.

As it went out on the air the following morning, the News Editor of the *Daily Express*'s northern office heard it on his car radio. Later in the morning, reporter Lynne Greenwood and photographer Phil Dunn came to see me. The 20th July issue of the *Express* carried a full-page feature – about me and with a piece about the scanner headlined: 'British, but we can't afford it'. The Fund was then at £31,000 but this national publicity doubled it within a month. It brought letters and donations from *Express* readers from all parts of Britain.

However, it did have one drawback. This was the first time any reference had been made in print to the fact that I was a terminal case. Now, I was *really* 'out in the open'. My little mother was most upset.

'What's all this about you being a dying woman? Where have they got that from?'

'Oh Mum, don't take any notice, it's only newspaper talk,' I lied.

'Well I think it's dreadful. They've no right to print a thing like that when it's not true!'

Oh heavens, how do I handle this?

'Look, love, give over. If I'm not worrying about it, why should you? We're *all* dying from the day we're born. Come on, let's put the kettle on and make a cuppa – I'm not dead yet!'

'Reporters make me sick,' declared my indignant Mum as she followed me into the kitchen. 'They take too many liberties!'

I started to giggle.

'How about *this* reporter? Do I make you sick?'

She glared at me.

'You've been a handful since the day you were born!'

I shook with laughter. 'What an epitaph!'

'Yes, but *you* wouldn't say someone was dying when they weren't. I'm not buying that paper any more! I've a good mind to ring and tell them so.'

I spent the rest of the morning trying to pacify her and my mind boggled at what the *Express*'s News Desk's reaction might be, should my irate mother give them a piece of her mind.

Forgive me, dear *Daily Express*, but for a few weeks you lost a reader. The same problem arose as other newspapers printed the truth, and each time I found it more and more difficult to reassure my mother. She took it out on my furniture, polishing it within an inch of its life. It was almost Christmas before I was able to tell her the true facts. By then, I was putting on weight and all signs of jaundice were gone.

But, at the time, running the house was a problem and I do not know how I would have managed without help. We have a four-bedroomed detached house which, before my illness, I had kept clean with a fairly systematic routine. At one time I would have thought nothing of setting to with wallpaper and paint and redecorating a room, getting a lot of satisfaction in the process. Now, with limited reserves of strength, housework was a nightmare. Even pushing and pulling the vacuum cleaner was beyond me, with the Titanic strapped to my chest. It's a frustrating business to know that jobs one has previously taken in one's stride, are now beyond one's capabilities. One day, when I had the house to myself, I sat looking at our sitting room with a critical eye and decided that the carpet needed shampooing

I filled a bucket with hot water and a liberal measure of carpet cleaner and got down on my knees to tackle it. I had scrubbed abour four square yards and my enthusiasm increased as the colour came up as good as the day it was laid. There was just one problem. The Titanic had sprung a leak and I had that sinking feeling. *Oh Lord, what have I done?*

An SOS to Marie, who happened to be on 'day off' and she came running across the road to give me a lecture and order me to bed. Threatening me with everything short of hell fire, she said I hadn't the sense I was born with and who did I think I was – Superwoman? She chastised me the whole time she was cleaning me up, swished the bedroom curtains with a fury that almost made them come off the rails; took the phone off the hook and forbade me to come downstairs for the rest of the day. When Geoff came home, I was on the receiving end of an even longer lecture. Phrases like 'damn fool thing to have done' and 'what's the good of a clean carpet if you land yourself back in the Christie?' sent me shrinking further under the sheets, feeling very like that little girl who had spent so much time at that desk in the school hall. I felt terrible, causing Geoff more worry, and even worse as I listened to him completing the cleaning of the carpet which I had left looking like the before-and-after pictures in the advert for a famous brand of soap powder. With paid domestic help only one morning a week, I don't know how I would have managed without my mother's competent assistance.

Hers is the kind of home where you could eat off the floor and shave in the patina of the furniture. To my mother, housework is not a series of chores, it's a matter of pride and joy. To me, it's a necessity if one is to maintain some standard of comfort and cleanliness. It's something which has to be done, but which takes up time I'd rather spend doing more creative things.

When I have been out on the 'Scanner Trail' Mother has often been here to answer the phone or receive callers. On my return, as well as a list of telephone messages, I'd find that she would have 'bottomed' the dining room or maybe the kitchen. On other occasions, she'd decide that my silver needed cleaning and would detail my father to come and see to it.

Geoff and Mike also became adept at doing chores which I would not have dreamed of asking them to do when I was fit. As far as the Fund was concerned the family backed me up in every way they could think of and the domestic front became a team effort. Our quiet, ordinary lives underwent an upheaval and, without it being put into words, the order of each day became Fund first, family second. I may have started the Appeal, but the Appeal took me and my family over.

I remember an occasion some years ago when Geoff and I and the children had visited the Brontë village, Haworth. Browsing round a craft shop, Geoff had bought himself an oilskin apron. It sported a picture of a jolly fat man in a white apron and hat. Underneath the picture were the words 'Le Chef'. The kids and I had burst out laughing when he came out of the shop with it.

'I don't know why on earth you've bought that – you can only boil an egg,' I had teased.

'Daddy makes beautiful beans on toast,' Helen had said, loyally.

At that time, boiled eggs and beans on toast were about the limits of Geoff's culinary exploits. Cancer and the 'Scanner Trail' changed all that. Now, he can cook most things. They may not be up to *cordon bleu* standard, but nobody is going to starve. And when you have become used to coming home from the office to find notes: 'dinner in oven', or 'chops/sausages/ham, etc. in fridge', and your wife is attending a function at the other end of the north-west, perhaps it is just as well!

The Appeal was keeping me increasingly busy as people rallied to the cause. I was attending more and more events clocking up endless miles on motorways. Fortunately, I like driving. I find it relaxing. I can sit behind the steering wheel of my car for hours on end yet if I have to stand for more than ten minutes I have to look round for a chair. I once sat down in the middle of a Mayor's speech.

It was either that, or fall at his feet. Fortunately, I knew this particular Mayor well enough to know that he wouldn't take it amiss. He was telling the audience about the first time he met me and how he had wondered how he should behave when his guest was a woman dying of cancer.

'I didn't expect to meet a lass who looked as ordinary and as normal as the rest of us,' said Councillor Jack Marsden of the Borough of South Ribble. 'Nor did I expect that she would enjoy a drink or a cigarette or that she would have a sense of fun, bordering on the ridiculous. Here was I, expecting to have to treat her like a piece of Dresden china and found that she seemed to have more stamina than any of us.'

Jack and his wife, Edith, did a great deal, during their year of office, to help the Appeal. Together with Robert and Helen Dickinson, Geoff and I enjoyed several evenings in their company, attending fund-raising events. Jack has a gregarious nature and a fund of anecdotes. He made sure that everyone enjoyed themselves, whether they liked it or not.

There have been occasions when I could *not* have sat down until the appropriate moment. Dignified, formal occasions, when, as well as having to stand, shifting my weight from one foot to the other, something has happened which I have found amusing and I have needed all my self-control to keep a sober expression. Like the time in a large hall, when the audience was asked to stand and the announcement was made, 'Ladies and gentlemen, the Mayor and Mayoress of X . . . Councillor and Mrs Y . . . and Mr and Mrs *Pat* Seed . . .'

I knew that if I had caught Geoff's eye, I would have been sunk . . . We progressed solemnly to our seats and sat down, after which, the assembled company also sat. I looked at Geoff and his expression said it all . .

'I didn't say it!' I whispered, 'Don't blame *me* . . .' I said, shaking with suppressed laughter. I am no advocate of Women's Lib – I like my bread buttered on both sides!

If travelling was no problem, arriving sometimes was! People, knowing their own districts with the familiarity of years of residence, would give me seemingly explicit directions for finding the places at which functions were to be held. They invariably ended by saying, 'You can't miss it,' to which I felt like replying, 'Do you want to bet?' for if anyone can get lost, it's me. I am the world's worst navigator. I must have done many petrol- and time-consuming detours before I hit on a different system. I arrange to meet my host or hostess at a mutually recognisable location – usually a pub – and they pilot me to wherever I am going. At least it means that I am there on time, instead of half an hour late.

Every day except Sunday, there is the mail. On rare evenings at home, I would be pounding the typewriter, sometimes until eleven thirty, or midnight.

'Isn't it time you called it a day?' my better half would suggest.

'I've only a couple more to answer and then I'm up-to-date.'

'How long do you think you're going to be able to keep up this pace? You know, you really should try to keep some sense of proportion. Surely those will wait until tomorrow?'

'There'll be more letters in the morning. I've got to try to keep abreast of them.' There were times when I felt like Canute, but I wouldn't have missed any of them.

Letters. Wonderful letters . . . letters to tug at my heart-strings. Letters full of goodwill, good wishes, affection and encouragement. Letters from the young, the old, the infirm. Letters to make me laugh and some to make me cry. Letters telling me how the senders had raised the money they'd enclosed – such as the contents of an office swear box. It seems the air in that office had been blue in support of what the staff considered to be a good cause. And in complete contrast, letters from people who had relatives dying of cancer and who didn't know how to cope. Such people could be at their wits' end and needed to get it off their chest to someone they thought would understand. To these people I could only offer my own recipe, 'One day at a time', plus the belief that Love itself is indestructible and never dies. Then there were many letters from the bereaved, sending donations in lieu of funeral flowers.

I am no use first thing in the morning. My biological clock is a slow starter. I can work until all hours of the night, but in the morning I am vulnerable. I learned not to open the mail until I had pulled myself together, for I never knew what it might contain.

One morning, at the bottom of the pile of letters was a packet. We collected trading stamps and the firm redeemed them for cash. It crossed my mind that the contents of the packet might be books of trading stamps. Among the letters was one from a young widow of twenty-seven, whose husband had recently died of cancer, leaving her with a little baby of eighteen months. 'Maybe if this money, which is instead of flowers for Bob's funeral, can be used to help other people, then his death will not seem such a completely wasteful thing . . .'

Poor little lass . . . my heart went out to her.

When I came to open the packet, the inner wrapping had on it the words 'anonymous gift' written in a shaky handwriting. Inside, there was £1,000 in £5 notes. I looked at the money in amazement and then I read again the letter from the young widow. It was too much. It was all too much. I sat and cried for almost half an hour. Blast this disease! Blast cancer! It had ruined this young girl's life and left that tiny child fatherless. Dear God, if ever I had any doubts about the rightness of what I was doing, this would have dispelled them.

'I'm not tough enough for this job,' I told myself, as I doused my face in cold water. As soon as my red swollen eyes looked reasonably near to normal, I went off to the bank with the generous gift from the unknown donor, for I never keep money in the house. It was an example of charity in the truest sense of the word.

I have kept every letter I have received throughout the Appeal. I treasure them. They have sustained me and encouraged me to carry on. They are a written witness to the essential goodness that is within most human beings. In doing something positive to help the Appeal, maybe the donors were helped as much as the Fund. In helping this particular fight against cancer, many people wrote to tell me that they felt they were 'hitting back' at the scourge which had deprived them of relatives and friends. To try to mention the names of all the people who have contributed would be to have this account read like the telephone directory. Nor can it be a comprehensive catalogue of fund-raising events, for it would need as many volumes as the *Encyclopaedia Britannica*. But among the myriad memories with which the 'Scanner Trail' has left me, certain incidents stand out in my mind as landmarks along the route, illustrating both the progress of the Appeal and the remarkable spirit which emerged as the need became increasingly recognised.

A letter arrived from a man in the Stockport area, telling me that he intended to walk the Pennine Way in aid of the Fund. The Pennine Way . . . 270 miles along the backbone of England, from Edale in Derbyshire to Kirk Yetholm on the Scottish border. Terry Arnold, ex-Royal Marine and former amateur boxing champion, intended to walk it in a week. A few years ago, Jos Naylor, who shins up and down Lakeland peaks like a mountain goat, had actually *run* the distance in three days, but nobody had walked the course in so short a time.

The *Manchester Evening News* had carried the story of Terry's proposed attempt and I said that the least I could do was to be at the finishing line to welcome him and thank him. Terry said that he expected to be at Kirk Yetholm at midday on Sunday, 17th July.

Ready for a break, Geoff and I decided to make a weekend of it. We hadn't had a holiday and a day or two 'away from it all' would do us good. On the Saturday, we set off up the M6 motorway, enjoying the Lakeland scenery, the glorious sunshine and just being alone together. As we drove along, peace and contentment were paramount. The mood was shattered as we approached the service station near Carlisle. The car exhaust had begun to make enough row to wake the dead. An unobtrusive arrival at the motorway workshop bay was impossible. Mechanics were working at full stretch, coping with the problems of holiday motorists. They couldn't help us. We drove at a noisy fifteen miles an hour into Carlisle, only to find that all the garages which supplied while-u-wait exhaust systems were shut and the owners had left the district. Eventually, we managed to buy a tin of adhesive bonding material which Geoff applied in liberal doses to the offending hole in the exhaust, which, needless to say, was in a most ungetatable part.

Then we headed gingerly in the direction of Kelso and

booked in for the night at an hotel in the main square.

Our twin-bedded room was nicely furnished in shades of pink, complete with a colour TV set and a tea-making machine. At right angles to the hotel was the Town Hall, whose clock recorded the passing of each quarter of an hour with ear-splitting monotony.

'Genevieve!'

'M'mm?'

'Genevieve. The film. Don't you remember? They had all that trouble with the car and when they finally got into their hotel room the town hall clock kept them awake all night. It starred Kenneth More, Dinah Sheridan and Kay Kendall.'

My tired spouse raised himself on one elbow and glared at me.

'Yes, well . . . if you're thinking of playing the trumpet, let me know and I'll move out!' With that he turned over and went to sleep, in spite of the town clock. As for me, it was the longest journey I'd made since I came out of hospital. I was so tired, I think I'd have slept on the clothes line.

The next morning, after a leisurely breakfast, we drove the few miles to the tiny village of Kirk Yetholm, nestling among the Border hills. It was just about noon when a tall blond man of splendid physique came off the fells, striding across the green, with a rucksack on his shoulders and looking as though he'd just had the dog out for its Sunday morning walk. There was no dog with him, but on his rucksack was a placard of Dayglo orange paper 'Pat Seed Cancer Appeal'. We took Terry into the Border Inn, where he downed several pints of ale with a speed which made me wonder if he'd got a hollow leg, or no 'clacker' in his throat. You can work up a magnificent thirst traipsing 270 miles over some of the roughest country in England. Terry also signed the book and claimed Wainwright's pint – donated by the author of *The Pennine Way* to all who completed the distance. The landlord told us that, as far as he knew, Terry's time was a walking record.

As well as being sponsored, Terry had handed out literature about the Appeal to other walkers and to proprietors of cafes and hostelries en route. His personal gear was of the minimum. He'd slept under the stars in a plastic survival bag and his primus stove was minute. As he recounted the various stages of his journey and told us of other groups of walkers he'd met with, it was apparent that the Pennine Way was a hard slog. Terry had derived a lot of pleasure and a sense of achievement from it, along with a crop of blisters which, he said, he had 'walked off'. How do you even begin to thank a man who has given up a week of his annual holiday and used his superb strength to further a cause you started? As he described the scenery to us, his affinity with nature and the countryside became obvious. I thanked him in the only way I knew:

FOR TERRY ARNOLD, WITH APPRECIATION AND GRATITUDE.

> Through forest glade of cool green shade,
> High mountain places, open spaces;
> Moorland tarns and farmstead barns,
> Cry of curlew, bleat of lambs
> What price now, the traffic jams?
>
> A packed rucksack, a fellside track,
> Sunshine, shadow, squally shower,
> The landscape changing by the hour;
> The silence of a starlit night,
> The glory of the dawn's first light.
>
> Where man and elements are one,
> Competing, yet in unison.
> Where one can find a peace of mind;
> Where body, heart and soul are free
> And Nature sings a rhapsody.

Just twelve months later, three teenage girls walked the Pennine Way from north to south. 'Nobody believed we would do it,' wrote Elizabeth, Sandra and Janice of Marple,

Cheshire. But they did and the Fund was £225 nearer the goal. Later still, a young man telephoned to say that he'd raised £300 by doing a sponsored walk and where had he to send the money? I gave him the information he required and asked him where he had walked.

'Oh, from Edale in Derbyshire to Hadrian's Wall.'

'What? The Pennine Way?'

'Yes.'

'That's a very tough walk, I'm told. Did you enjoy it?'

'No, not particularly,' replied Neil Taylor of Newcastle under Lyne.

'Oh, what a shame. What happened?'

'I had a broken leg.'

'Good heavens! Did you break it on the walk?'

'No, I was doing some mountaineering about three weeks before. There was a bit of bone lodged in the joint. It was strapped up, but I could still walk on it, so I decided to go ahead.'

Aren't some people incredible?

Young people have done some remarkable things. A group of Young Farmers from Read in East Lancashire decided they'd do a sponsored wheelchair push from Blackpool to Burnley. With four girls in wheelchairs borrowed from a local hospital and eight strapping lads as the pushers, they hired a Dormobile as a back-up vehicle. The cost of hiring the van should have been £36 but when the owner knew why they wanted it, he reduced the charge to £6, even putting in £4 worth of free petrol in the tank. The Dormobile was piled high with chicken legs, other farmhouse goodies and enough homemade soup to float the *Queen Mary*. At ten o'clock on a Friday night, they set off from Blackpool. Several times, they were stopped by police who wanted to know what they were up to and, I'm told, several pairs of socks ended up in litter bins en route for Burnley. But they hadn't finished at that. They retraced their steps and came to Garstang, where I met them on Saturday lunchtime and we all had a drink together in the Royal Oak Hotel. Then they pushed all the way back to Burnley again and blow me, if they didn't go to a disco at night! Where they found the energy to dance after such a feat – or should it be 'feet'? – I will never know. Some weeks later, Julé Hayward and I met the intrepid Young Farmers in their local at Read and they gave us the cheque for their sponsor money, over £1,000.

In September, we held a Garden Fête in the grounds of the staff club at the Christie. This was opened by Brian Redhead and was very successful. Hospital staff provided entertainment, stalls were manned by some of the branch committees of the Fund, of which we now had more than thirty, and the first prize of the raffle was a football signed by Sir Matt Busby and the stars of Manchester United. Earlier, I had written to their Secretary, Mr Leslie Olive, with whom I had been at school, asking if the club could help in any way. Les had kindly sent the football. It was the first of several to be raffled in aid of the Fund and this one raised £800, making the afternoon s proceeds about two and a half thousand pounds and the Fund total over £90,000. As the money mounted up, so did my sense of responsibility increase. I needed help. I needed a Central Committee of the Fund.

I needed a group of eminent people who would lend their names and their varying expertise to be a policy making team. But who to ask? I pondered on this question for a long time before I decided on the people to approach.

Mr Michael Fitzherbert Brockholes, whose family have lived at Claughton Hall, near Garstang, for several centuries is a gentleman held in the highest esteem by our local population. He is a Lancashire County Councillor, Chairman of Garstang Magistrates and is also Vice Lord Lieutenant of Lancashire. He knew me as a local reporter and a local resident. He also knew of the Appeal and its objectives. When

I asked him if he would be a member of my Central Committee, he very kindly offered to help me in any way he could. I wrote to Sir William Downward, Lord Lieutenant of Greater Manchester, who readily offered his assistance. I wanted a member of my own profession, who would appreciate the need for progressive publicity and was thankful when Mr Douglas Emmet, editor of the *Manchester Evening News*, accepted my invitation. On such a committee, I wanted someone who knew me personally. I could think of no person I would rather have than one of our oldest friends, Mr Roy Fisher, Chairman of the Chorley Magistrates bench. Roy and my husband had been friends long before either of them had met their respective wives. The twosome then became a foursome and as Roy and Kay's two daughters and Michael and Helen arrived on the scene, it became an eightsome, with both pairs of adults standing as Godparents to one of the others' children. Shared holidays together when the children were small and a close association over the years has ensured that our friendship with the Fisher family is the kind that lasts a lifetime. By profession, Roy is a consultant architect – just the man to keep an eye on plans for a scanner building. Together with Christie doctors – Radiotherapist Ian Todd, Principal Physicist David Greene, Diagnostician Brian Eddleston and Treasurer Mr Geoffrey Ball, this was the nucleus of the Central Committee, which first met on 3rd October. Later, we enlisted the help of Mr R. Calderwood, Town Clerk and Chief Executive of Manchester; Mr David Wilson, President of the Manchester Chamber of Commerce and Mrs Peggy Keats, Secretary and Treasurer of the Lady Julia Holt Women's Trust Fund.

Sir William was appointed chairman, with Mr Brockholes as vice chairman and, in preparation for the Trust Deed to be registered with the Charity Commissioners, four Trustees were appointed: Sir William Downward, Mr Roy Fisher, Dr Todd and Dr Eddleston.

All of these people were, and are, heavily committed with their own professional pursuits and with their individual community and charitable activities. One of the biggest head-aches with such a committee is to find mutually convenient dates when members can meet. But then, they do say, if you want something doing, ask people who are busy – the others never have the time. It was a weight off my mind to know that I had such a team behind me.

October also brought another kind of relief. In late September, the Titanic started giving trouble. I developed an infection which failed to respond to antibiotics. (Oh hell, what's going wrong now?) The Christie surgeon who had performed the operation in January said that my body was trying to reject it because it no longer had any use for it. It was a foreign body my own body did not want.

'You'd better come in for a day and we'll remove it for you.'

Immediately, I got all up-tight and apprehensive. After all these months, the thing was a part of me. Would they give me an anaesthetic? A reassuring smile, together with the reply that an anaesthetic wasn't necessary for such a simple procedure. *Simple?* For all I knew, half my inside might come out along with that rubber tubing – and if it did, I didn't want to know about it! I was given an intravenous dose of a tranquilliser before being wheeled down to theatre. At the end of a long day of performing operations, the surgeon must have been tired, but he still had patience with the shivering bundle of nerves on the trolley. For a few minutes, he chatted about the Appeal and then: 'We'll just remove the dressing . . .' he murmured. Like a conjuror producing a rabbit out of a hat, he lifted the dressing into the air, complete with eighteen inches of drain tube attached. I hadn't felt a thing.

Was this what I'd made such a fuss about? I felt all kinds of a fool. But oh, the freedom. To be able to move more easily . . . to be able to wallow in a warm bath whenever I felt like it, instead of waiting until it was convenient for Marie to fix the Titanic. It was sheer luxury to be able to turn over in bed without that cube pressing into my chest. I hadn't realised just how restrictive it had been. 'What happens if I need it again?' I had asked the surgeon.

'Oh, we'll soon put it back for you.'

Not if I can help it! I thought.

And as the months went by, I was putting on weight. I had progressed from a size twelve, through size fourteen and by the time the Fund was one year old, I was to be back to my normal weight, back to being a size-sixteen-struggling-not-to-be-a-size-eighteen. Clothes which I had pushed to the back of my wardrobe because they hung on me like sacks, were called upon for further service. Somewhat regretfully, the size twelves went to a jumble sale. Pity. I'd enjoyed being slim, even though friends had told me 'It just isn't you.' However, I gave myself a lecture on getting my priorities right. I was ALIVE, wasn't I? That's all that mattered. Every day was a bonus and I gave thanks for it. I didn't look like anyone's idea of a dying woman. With my tanned complexion and rosy cheeks puffed up to nearly twice their normal size by drugs, I was beginning to feel that I should apologise for looking so healthy. Then I told myself not to be an idiot! If I looked the picture of health, then I was a credit to the Christie. To those who equated the hospital with doom, gloom and death. I was a good advert for what the staff of the hospital could achieve. But for them, I would have been six feet under the sod, months ago. Here was another way to allay fear. OK – so I didn't know how long it would last, but every day I lived was a day I wouldn't have had but for the skills of the Christie doctors.

And whenever a man or a woman told me that they had been a patient of the Christie, maybe ten or fifteen years ago, and were now cured, I would say: 'If you are one of Christie's cures, then go and shout it from the housetops. *You* are just the kind of person who could do a great deal to remove fear and encourage others to seek help in time.' Some said they didn't like it known that they had had cancer. To these people, I said that in sheer thankfulness for their own good fortune, it was a way in which they could be of service to their fellow human beings, far too many of whom didn't realise that many forms of cancer are curable – if *only* they are dealt with in time.

On the other hand, there have been a number of people who have wanted to tell me every last detail of a relative's case history before dying of cancer. If telling me gave them some sort of relief, then I was prepared to listen. Still more would describe their own symptoms and ask me if I thought they had cancer. I could only recommend that if they had any doubts at all, they should seek the advice of their doctor, either to have their mind put at rest or to obtain the earliest possible treatment. When some persisted, 'Yes, but what do *you* think it is?' I would tell them firmly, 'I'm not a doctor. I'm not qualified to diagnose. You wouldn't ask a bricklayer to mend your television, would you?'

Some people asked, 'How can you be so bright and cheerful when you know you could die at any time?'

'Look, dear, you could be knocked down by a car, be involved in a train or plane crash tomorrow. Does that thought worry you?'

'No.'

'Exactly. I could die of cancer tomorrow – but that's *tomorrow*, not today. Today, I'm reasonably well and I'm happy. If the worst happens tomorrow, that's when I'll worry about it.' And it was true. My 'one day at a time' philosophy worked. It was bringing me through the barrier of fear to an acceptance that worry accomplishes not one damn thing. And because each day was a bonus it added a quality to life where colours seemed brighter, perception was keener. In those April days of 1976, I had lain in bed watching the cherry tree outside my bedroom window. I had watched the first buds appear and grow to full flower, before cascading a pink filigree of petals on to the lawn. And because I thought I'd never see it blossom again, I appreciated it so much more. The pleasure it gave me was immeasurable and I no longer took it for granted. In full bloom, it was like a Cinderella dressed for the ball, emerging from the drab brown branches of winter. I've watched my cherry tree blossom twice since then and felt just the same about it. Before cancer, I'd probably have thought the tree very pretty – and moaned about the mess the petals made as they fell. Not any more.

If cancer has brought me pain, suffering and the knowledge that I'm not likely to get a telegram from the Monarch congratulating me for having lived for a hundred years, it has also given me an appreciation of the real value of life and the knowledge that the most priceless things are not those bought with money. Money cannot buy the love of one human for another, or affection, comradeship or goodwill. And in the course of the Appeal, in the two years since I was told I'd 'had it' I have probably seen more of the good side of human nature than any one person has a right to expect to see in an entire lifetime. For that, it is almost worth having cancer.

'Look, love, get your diary and I'll get mine. Let's see if we can find a weekend when both of us are free and let's clear off somewhere.'

'Where d'you fancy going?' Geoff asked.

'Quite frankly, I don't care, as long as we get a bit of a break. I'm ready for one and I know you are, too!'

For one reason and another, we hadn't managed a summer holiday. The only break we'd had was the weekend in the Border Country, when we went to meet Terry after his marathon walk. That's how, on the morning of Friday, 11th November, we came to set off in the pale, late autumn sunshine, in the direction of the Yorkshire Dales. Had we known it, we couldn't have picked a more disastrous weekend. But at that time, ignorance was bliss.

We motored along, in no particular hurry, with Bonnie Boy on my knee and our case and his basket on the back seat of Geoff's car. We enjoyed a leisurely lunch at the Cross Keys at East Marton and by late afternoon we arrived at the Bluebell Hotel, Kettlewell, where we booked in for the night. We had an excellent dinner and spent the evening in the bar, chatting with the landlord and the regulars. Bonnie came in for a lot of attention, but he took exception to a motor cyclist who came into the pub in his leathers. On the following day we intended to drive to York, to have a look round the ancient city and visit the Minster.

But, as they say, the best-laid plans . . . this time, it wasn't the car that went wrong, it was the weather. The walls of the Bluebell are about six feet thick and for centuries they have withstood all that the furious elements have thrown at them. Although we realised it was a wild and stormy night, we were not aware of what was happening on the Lancashire coast.

After breakfast on Saturday morning, we packed our belongings into the car. It was raining and the wind was an icy blast. I was beginning to wonder whether a weekend away was such a good idea, after all, when a news bulletin on the car radio confirmed that for us it certainly was not. Winds in the Irish sea are somewhat unpredictable. During the late hours of Friday night and the early hours of Saturday morning and with little or no warning, storm-force gales had veered due west, whipping up an expected 29-feet spring tide by another 7-feet surge and hurling it with fearful impact inland. It caused severe flooding and widespread damage to large areas of the Lancashire coast. In deeper water off shore, waves varied from 16 to 23 feet. Normally adequate sea defences had been unable to cope with the monstrous waves.

Many people were flooded out and were temporarily homeless. Huge blocks of concrete were tossed about like pebbles. Farmland was inundated by the sea, cattle died and many farmers lost a lifetime's work in just a few short, nightmare hours. For hundreds of square miles, the cruel sea created a havoc unparalleled for sixty years. The misery and devastation of that night was a natural disaster which was to take months to put right.

My husband is the land drainage area engineer, Rivers Division, for the North-West Water Authority. We headed for home as fast as the car would take us. The staffs of the Water Authority, the local authorities and all emergency services worked around the clock. These were some of the biggest tides of the year and more storm-force westerly gales were forecast. For the next couple of weeks, I only saw Geoff when he came home to snatch a couple of hours' sleep before going out again.

Compared with what some people had lost, a weekend away was a mere nothing. And on Monday, I was back on the 'Scanner Trail' again, with several engagements in the Oldham and Rochdale areas.

The Appeal was leaving me little time for journalism. I was sending in less and less copy and it worried me. There just weren't enough hours in the day. I was retained by two evening papers to report Garstang area news and they had a right to expect far better coverage than I was now giving. When I broached the matter, the editors of both papers were very understanding. 'Don't worry. We know what you're trying to do. Keep up the good work. Send us whatever you can.' We arranged that if I couldn't cover a job myself, I'd pass it on to news desk as information and, if necessary, they'd have staff reporters deal with it. It was the best I could do and I salved my conscience with the thought that the Appeal itself was creating plenty of human interest stories and plenty of column inches about the things people were doing in support of it. I missed my work and my income had taken a nose dive. But the 'Scanner Trail' had to take precedence.

Meanwhile, the Fund's solicitors were getting to work on the Trust Deed. A couple of preliminary drafts were prepared and discussed by the Central Committee before it was finalised and submitted to the Charity Commissioners. This, in itself, proved to be a cliffhanger.

October and November is the time of the year when most firms make their donations to charity and many will not contribute unless the charity is registered. I wanted to send a letter of appeal to North-West Commerce, Industry and Trade. Some weeks before, I'd ordered a guide to north-west firms at our local stationers and it still hadn't arrived. In desperation, I rang the publishing firm. No, the book was not yet ready.

'Have you got your galley-proofs?'

I explained why I wanted them and they were most co-operative. The administration office at the Christie sent a hospital car over to the firm's premises, borrowed the galley proofs and one of the secretaries worked late to photocopy the lot – nearly a hundred and eighty pages of them, containing the names and addresses of 7,000 north-west firms. The next day, they were returned to the publishers.

Our local printer had my letter of appeal, over a facsimile signature, set up in type. All we were waiting for was the charity registration number. Daily, I rang our solicitors. 'Has it come yet?' or, 'If it doesn't come soon, we're going to miss the boat.'

On 28th November, Miss Anne Dixon, articled clerk of Messrs Ingham, Clegg and Crowther rang me to say that she'd telephoned the Charity Commissioners and they'd given her the number. 'It's come through. Your number if 506996 – you can go ahead.' Call to Colin Cross: 'Here's the number.

Slot that line of type in – and *please* 7,000 of those letters as quick as you can.'

'I know,' said Colin. 'You want them yesterday, as usual!' I chuckled down the telephone.

'The day before that, if you can manage it!'

Meanwhile, with the help of our two local papers, *The Courier* and the *Garstang Guardian*, I had enlisted the help of about forty volunteers, all of whom were prepared to spare a few hours or more. Mostly ladies, they were members of local WIs, Mothers' Unions, Ladies Circle, Inner Wheel, my fellow Soroptimists, plus one or two older girls of the Youth Club. In the evenings, one or two men turned up, including my ever-patient husband. Cabus Village Hall Committee lent us the hall for free and we developed an urgent conveyor-belt system.

Those with neat clear handwriting or who possessed typewriters, addressed envelopes; others folded letters and another group put them in the envelopes. I cut Geoff's best car sponge into about eight pieces (promising faithfully to buy him a new one), and still more folk stuck down flaps and stuck on stamps – 7,000 of them. It took us three afternoons and evenings at the village hall and a group of us finished the job at our house on the morning of the fourth day.

Our local sorting office must have wondered what had hit them, for the letters filled six large Post Office sacks. But, like everyone else, they rallied to the occasion, even sending a van to collect them. At the end of it all, we all felt as though we didn't want to see another envelope as long as we lived. But the task was accomplished, and only just in time.

A few days later, the replies started to come in. An army of volunteers helped me yet again, this time to acknowledge the donations. Only a small percentage of firms said that they were unable to contribute, mainly because they were now subsidiaries of larger companies whose charitable donations were handled by their head offices, usually in other parts of the country. Another small percentage of my letters were returned to sender, because the firms had gone out of business. Many had been unable to compete with the larger concerns and some had succumbed to the economic climate of the times.

But, by and large, the response was magnificent. Donations varied from £5 to £1,000 and behind the business-like replies enclosing their contributions, one could sense a warmth, a sympathetic regard. Those who were unable to contribute refused with seemingly genuine regret and in some cases, gave the address of their parent company.

I hoped the Fund would reach £200,000 by the end of the year. Instead, it topped £300,000. Here was I, with my batteries constantly in need of recharging and with my engine only firing on three cylinders, driving myself harder than at any other period of my life. It had been a mammoth task. It had left me and some of my willing helpers, without whom it would have been utterly impossible, in a state of near collapse and with no desire at all to write our own Christmas cards.

Ruefully, I decided that there was one phrase in that Trust Deed which was not appropriate. Although it was necessary to meet legal requirements, I was referred to as 'The Retiring Trustee'.

If ever there was a misnomer, *that was it!*

6

The Bright Star

Combine the robust, rapier-sharp wit of his native Liverpool
with a sense of the ridiculous, plus an ability to establish an
easy rapport with his audience from the moment he comes on
stage and you have a comedian of star rating. Add to this a
fine melodious singing voice – with several chart toppers and
some gold and silver recording discs to prove it – and it's no
wonder that Ken Dodd has been described as the comedian
people don't mind missing the last bus home for. He can have
an audience aching with laughter. Seconds later, he's soothing
them with one of the sentimental ballads he's made entirely
his own. 'Tears for Souvenirs' alone sold over two million
singles. As one of Britain's top-flight comics, Ken Dodd can
command a four-figure fee for a one-night stand. He might
be forgiven if he spent much of his time abroad, keeping his
'brass' in his own pocket or in a Swiss bank account, instead
of handing over much of what he earns to the Tax Man. That
isn't the nature of the man. For Doddy, Britain is the finest
country in the world and it has his love and loyalty. As well
as making a considerable impact on, and adding a whole new
facet to Show Biz, Ken has placed his own indelible imprint
on the English vocabulary. Who, for instance, had heard of

words such as 'dis-cum-knockerated' or 'plumpshushful' before his rise to stardom? Yet when he uses them on stage, his audiences know exactly what he means.

Though his name has been a household word for more than two decades, few people realise that Knotty Ash is not just the home of the Diddy men or a figment of his fertile imagination. It is a real place on the outskirts of Liverpool. It's where he was brought up and where he still lives in the family home. Ken Dodd has appeared on the bill of the Royal Variety Show seven times; he's entertained at the Royal Household Christmas Party; he's appeared on television more times than he can count and he's trodden the boards of every stage of any consequence throughout Britain. When one tries to pinpoint what makes this man so popular, one starts by thinking of his talent, his superb sense of timing, his seemingly boundless energy and a whole miscellany of other qualities. Then one realises that behind that whimsical buffoonery, there is a very sincere, caring human being. His humour is based on first-rate observation of human behaviour and he uses it to make us laugh at ourselves. For the essential characteristic of Ken is his genuine love of people. Without always being consciously aware of it, audiences instinctively recognise this and they respond accordingly. Of all the media, his first love is live theatre where footlights are no barrier between him and his audience. He's spent much of his time and effort *and* his own financial resources in successful attempts to save many of the country's provincial theatres from permanent closure. For Ken, theatres are not just places to work. He regards them as an integral part of our national heritage and he spares no personal effort to ensure that as many as possible are preserved. That is why, in late 1977, he speculated £100,000 of his own money to try to save the Palace Theatre, Manchester. It was an enterprise which paid off. Full houses of appreciative audiences ensured that the Ken Dodd Laughter Show, staged during the six weeks Christmas season, was successful. They came from all over the north-west and, as usual, they got value for money. So did Manchester. The outcome was that a Trust was formed to secure that theatre's future.

Few comedians can come to the front of the stage at close on midnight and say to the audience, 'Have you had enough? D'you give in?' The reply is always a loud chorus of 'NO!' They'd sit there just as long as he was prepared to stay on stage.

I had seen Ken many times, long before I met him in person. A favourite with Blackpool audiences, his summer season at the Opera House was always a sellout, with local residents competing for seats along with the influx of holiday visitors.

I've enjoyed many a night there and come home with my ribs aching, trying to remember at least some of the jokes which seem to pour out of him as quickly as water going over Niagara.

During the week including Wednesday, 12th October 1977, Ken was appearing at the Park Hall Leisure Centre, Charnock Richard. Robert and Helen Dickinson had arranged a charity night for the Fund. With Ken's reputation as a crowd puller, they thought it would not only give people a good night out, but it would help to swell our coffers. On both counts, I was delighted and, sure enough, Park Hall was packed. Before Ken came on stage, we went backstage to meet him. During the conversation I nodded in the direction of the door by which he'd entered.

'Is that your dressing room?'

'Yes.'

'Would you mind if I had a word with you in private?'

'Surely.'

In his dressing room he asked what he could do for me.

In as few words as possible, I told him about myself and what I was hoping to accomplish. I asked him if he would consider being a Patron of the Fund.

'What I'm asking of you, is that you will lend your name and your prestige to this Appeal. I didn't want to ask you in front of other people in case you would prefer to say "no". I know how heavily committed you are.'

'How much will it cost me? You see, I've just sunk a tidy sum into the show I'm putting on to try to save the Manchester Palace.'

'I'm not asking you for money. If you will lend your name to this Appeal, anything else you choose to contribute would be entirely up to you.'

For a long moment he looked at me. Then he took my hand.

'Anything I can do to help you, you've only to ask. If I can do it, I will. If I can't, I will say so.'

Ken is no stranger to the cancer problem. Only a few months before he had lost his fiancée, Anita Boutin. Surgery had failed to save her and she had died of a brain tumour. There was nothing I could tell Ken about the heartbreak and misery of losing a loved one through this scourge that he didn't already know for himself. He also knew the value of the scanner.

In the course of the next few months, I realised that I'd not only gained a staunch ally, but a friend. He did innumerable 'free' shows in various venues up and down the north-west in aid of the Fund. I wasn't able to attend all of them, but I must have sat through Ken's act at least seven times in as many months and such is the calibre of the man that I laughed just as much at each successive performance. Personal worries fade into the background or are entirely forgotten when he is on stage. I remember remarking on this, saying: 'It must give you a lot of satisfaction, knowing you can do this for people?'

He thought for a moment and then said, 'Yes, I suppose it does.' Then, with that irrepressible humour that's never far from the surface, he added with a grin: 'Of course, I like the money as well!'

'Oh, get off with you! If money were your God you'd have been a tax exile years ago.'

And when, somewhat diffidently, he replied, 'I just regard money as a measure of success.' He was speaking no more and no less than the truth.

Ken's organist, Stan Clarke, and the other members of his entourage say he's a great bloke to work with. I have no doubt that this is so. Show Business is exacting and exhausting. As well as fame and being on the receiving end of a lot of adulation, stars like Ken Dodd put in a lot of hard graft. No matter how much you may enjoy it, when you've given all you've got on stage, you come off it feeling drained. The shows Ken did for me were on his days or nights off – times when he could have been at home, putting his feet up. All he asked in return was a donation for Merseyside's Clatterbridge Hospital, for the provision of new laboratories. He has put in just as much effort, done just as many free performances to help Clatterbridge as he has for my Appeal. To such an extent that it's a wonder the lad hasn't found himself in a hospital bed instead of working to help those already in them. He invited me as his guest to attend the 'sod cutting ceremony' on the day the building work began on the site for Clatterbridge's laboratories. Few people see the serious side of Ken Dodd. That day was no exception. After several formal speeches by officials of the hospital and those of various other organisations, Ken was asked to cut the first sod. As one would expect, it was something of a pantomime. No symbolic blades of grass and an ounce or two of earth removed in sober fashion on the end of a polished steel spade! The tool for this job was an earth moving machine.

Ken got into the cab and the regular driver tried to give some off-the-cuff instructions. However, it obviously takes more than one lesson before you are an expert at handling one of these weighty vehicles. The machine didn't seem to know in which direction it was expected to traverse and the long arm with the shovel on the end of it swung about in menacing fashion. The overall impression was that of an inebriated Dalek and as Ken was the only one of the assembled company wearing a protective helmet, discretion became the better part of valour and we all retreated to a safe distance from where we could watch and laugh in safety.

It was on this day that I first met Kay Kelly. Kay and I have much in common, for she is a cancer patient of Clatter-bridge Hospital. Like me, she has been told that it's 'only a matter of time' and similarly, she's determined to do what she can for the hospital. We had spoken on the telephone and when Ken invited me to the sod-cutting ceremony, I asked if I could bring Kay along. I introduced them to each other and they swopped telephone numbers. Also there, were journalists of the *Liverpool Daily Post* and *Echo* and other local papers. I asked them if they would give Kay every possible help.

Ken and I see things in the same way inasmuch as neither of us sees any need for rivalry between the two Appeals. The Christie needs a scanner and Clatterbridge needs new labora-tories; it's all part of the same fight against disease and both Appeals need all the help they can muster. To see it otherwise is to be guilty of small mindedness. I have also had people write to me from other parts of the country who have wanted to start appeals for scanners in their own areas. I have tried to be as helpful as possible. The starting point must always be to ascertain whether the hospital would welcome such a gift and the relevant Area Health Authority approves of it.

I had asked Ken if he could spare the time to visit patients in the Christie with me during the pre-Christmas period and on 22nd December, he did just that. I had put on a bright red dress with a gold belt in an attempt to look Christmassy.

As we walked up the stairs to one of the upper floors, he

asked me, 'Who are you supporting? Liverpool or Manchester United?' (both teams' football kit is red).

'Listen, going up these stairs is taking me all my time to support myself!'

He did a great deal to boost the morale of those patients who would be spending their Christmas in the hospital. He signed autographs by the dozen, much to the delight of patients and staff. One elderly lady said to me: 'He talked to us as though we really *mattered*. He didn't just walk through the ward so that we only got a glimpse of him.'

We spent a long time in the children's ward. To see little children, too ill and too lethargic to care what day of the week it is, never mind three days before Christmas, is one of the saddest sights on earth. Equally harrowing are the anxious young parents, sitting one either side of each bed. There were several little patients like this, including one little boy from Liverpool. Ken spent a lot of time talking to this little man and his Mum and Dad. Other children, who were out-patients, had come into the ward for the Christmas party which was to take place later in the afternoon. Some of them, because of the treatment they were having, had lost their hair. The little girls overcame this by wearing headscarves, knotted fashionably in gipsy style, but some of the little boys didn't have this advantage. Eventually, their hair would grow again when their course of treatment was over.

I came out of that ward with a lump in my throat the size of a duck egg. Some of those children would get better, some of them wouldn't. I felt the familiar fury and frustration against cancer, which would make some of these little lives of such brief duration. Whenever I feel myself flagging, it is little ones like these I think of. But even though you could weep buckets, you paint a smile on your face along with the lipstick.

In another ward we came across a young man, sitting in the chair next to his bed. His hand was taped to a saline drip feed and from his chest protruded a drain tube. It looked all too familiar.

Ken sat on the edge of the bed and tried to make conversation with him. The young man answered in monosyllables, contributing hardly anything to the conversation. His morale was obviously at a very low ebb and his lack of response began to get embarrassing.

'You're on a drip feed, aren't you?' I said.

He nodded.

'And that's a drain tube sticking out of your chest, isn't it?'

'Yes.'

'Well, will you take a look at me? This time last year, I was in exactly your position. I know just how you feel, for I've been through it. The doctors will do everything they can to make you well again, but you've got to do your part as well.'

'How d'you mean?'

'I mean that you are part of the team. You have to fight every inch of the way and *never give in*. Come on, you can do it!'

After a few minutes we left him and Ken said: 'Did you see the difference in that lad? His shoulders lifted about three inches. You did far more for him than I did.'

'Maybe. Let's hope it lasts.'

I didn't see that young man again. I don't know if he got better or not. But if, for one day, his spirits were lifted, then time had not been wasted. Finally, we went into the administration office where the staff had laid on sherry and biscuits. Old time music hall artiste Nat Jackley and his wife were there. As Ken was chatting to them, Pam Barber, the clerk who handles the Appeal mail which comes to Christie, said to me: 'I've just had a bank manager on the phone. One of his clients wants to give you £40,000.'

'£40,000! My stars! Who is it?'

'He wouldn't say. His client wishes to remain anonymous.

He was asking for particulars of the Appeal at this stage, but said that he would contact us within the next few days.'

'But that's marvellous! What a Christmas present.'

I thought of those little ones up in the Children's Ward whom we had visited just a short while ago and I could have hugged the unknown donor. £40,000 brought the scanner so much nearer. On the last day of 1977, this generous cheque arrived at the Christie and I tried to express my gratitude, sending my letter to the manager of the bank for him to forward to his client. Some days later I received a reply. The letter came without the sender's signature or address. The writer said that totally unexpectedly and right out of the blue, the family had found themselves on the receiving end of a large sum of money. Having catered for the needs of those nearest to them, they thought it would be little short of criminal to sit on money that could be used to help others. For a long time, they had considered what they should do with it and had decided that the Appeal should benefit. In my letter of thanks I had mentioned the children in the Christie and the donor commented: 'If only *one* such family can be relieved of this anxiety and face the future with confidence with their child because of this money, then it is worth every penny. It comes with the heartfelt sincerity of one Lancashire family who wish you well and your Appeal every success.'

I have many souvenirs of the Appeal which are treasures beyond price. This letter is one of them. I shall keep it as long as I live. When news of this splendid donation made the headlines, there was much speculation as to who it could be. Many people reckoned they knew who it was. They were all wrong. Although I know from which area of Lancashire it comes, I would not dream of trying to find out the identity of this family, for I have too much respect for their wish to remain anonymous.

Another souvenir arrived on 23rd December. It was from a primary school near Blackpool, enclosing the cheque which was the proceeds of their carol service. It came with a card, made of orange coloured school paper, folded in concertina fashion and which opened out to two feet long. Each child in the school had drawn a little cut-out figure, coloured it and pasted it on the card, writing his or her name underneath. Some of them had added a kiss. On the front, it said: To Pat Seed from all of us at Stalmine School. The tears I'd held back at the Christie in the Children's Ward on the previous day, now overflowed. Here, if only they knew it, were children helping children. I am not ashamed of my tears. I will fight with everything I've got for this cause in which I believe and I will work all the hours God sends. But there have been some aspects of the Appeal which have been a great emotional strain. It's not the work, the travelling or the fourteen-, fifteen- and sometimes sixteen-hour day that I put in which undermines me. It is the sheer undiluted kindness of folk. The very many examples of goodwill, of humanity at its best, which have reduced me to tears. Unlike cancer, kindness is an amiable disease. In support of the Fund it has been nurtured with constant practice by a great many people. It has spread like a benevolent plague. I suppose tears are a safety valve. I cannot listen to Ken's hit song 'Tears For Souvenirs' without realising that tears are among my souvenirs.

'I'm going to enjoy this Christmas. I don't remember a thing about the last one, so I'm going to make up for it, this time around.' The thought was accompanied by a sense of incredulity, for to be honest, I hadn't expected to see another Christmas. However, all the more reason for celebrating. Christmas really began for me on Saturday, 17th December. Every year, the Blackpool Corps of the Salvation Army puts on a Festival of Carols and Christmas Music in the Opera House. The collection during the interval is donated to charity and this year, the charity was the Appeal Fund.

The Salvation Army are noted for their joyous and tuneful

music and tonight's programme was no exception. Every one of the theatre's 3,000 seats were occupied.

It was a very moving experience for me when baritone Brian Parkinson sang one of my carols. The tune is familiar. Originally a Russian folk melody, it was first sung in this country by the Red Army Choir. Later, as 'The Carnival Is Over', it was a hit record for the New Seekers some years ago. I had written some words to it for my Sunday School children, which were intended to convey that the Christmas story was only the opening chapter of the story of Jesus, and that it should be seen in the context of the whole story.

BRIGHTEST STAR

Brightest star of highest heaven
Shining radiance o'er the night;
Angel choirs of glory singing
As the sky is filled with light.

Heralding a Saviour Shepherd,
Come to earth to save His sheep;
But for now, a helpless infant
In His mother's arms, asleep.

For a while, a carefree childhood,
With its pleasure and its fun;
But this child of gentle Mother
Is the Lord God's only Son.

Not just yet will sorrow find Him;
Not just yet, the pain and grief
Of rejection by a people
Full of pride and unbelief.

Born to save our human frailty,
Came this life of perfect love;
Priceless gift to us, His children
From the Lord of heaven above.

At this joyful Christmas season,
So the star will shine once more
With its message, the renewal
Of His promise, ever sure.

Major Taylor told the audience that he hoped to be able to give me a cheque for £300 for the Fund but that would depend entirely on how generous they were prepared to be. What in fact was collected, was £600. The stage of the Opera House is the largest in Europe. I knew that towards the end of the evening's programme, I would have to walk on to that stage to say some words of thanks. The thought terrified me. I sat in the front row of the dress circle for two hours, with my tummy tied in knots and my knees knocking. When Major Taylor did invite me on stage, it was overwhelming to see all those people in the stalls, the circle and the balcony. Then suddenly, I could feel their goodwill towards me. It was almost a tangible thing. There was a warmth coming towards me and I thought, 'what am I worrying about? They are all my friends.' and I was able to talk to them naturally as if we were all sitting round the fireside, having a nice cosy cup of tea. One tends to forget that every one of those 3,000 people, is just one person.

I would never want to earn my living on the stage. Goodness knows what I could do to amuse an audience, anyway. But it did give me some insight into the pull of Show Business. For people like Ken Dodd and the stars of the entertainment world, such audiences are the breath of life itself.

But not to my husband! Getting Geoff to wear a fancy dress costume is just about as unlikely as getting the devil to Holy Communion.

Just before Christmas 1977, John and Brenda Wilding, owners of Th'Owd Tithebarn Licensed Restaurant in Garstang, decided to hold an 'Olde English Nite' in aid of the Fund. The stipulation was 'no admittance unless wearing a costume of no later period than the 1920s'.

The restaurant itself is the result of a mammoth do-it-yourself exercise by John, who had bought the derelict tithebarn and renovated and refurbished it, using natural materials. At one end is a huge open fireplace which will burn a dozen or more outsize logs at a time. From the rafters hang a collection of antique agricultural implements. A long centre table, which was once the back of a church pew was laden on 'the Nite' with whole hams, sides of beef, half lambs and a variety of other succulent foods all presented in old English style and all of which had been donated.

What to wear? A friend had lent me a medieval dress and had offered Geoff a Cavalier outfit. The latter was made to fit a man of about five feet ten inches tall. Geoff is six feet three. As well as using all my powers of persuasion, I had a practical problem. Out came the sewing machine. By hook and several safety pins I managed to make it fit. Silver tinfoil buckles for his black shoes, white tights, red velvet breeches, a frilled lace shirt, a swirling red cloak, plus a wide brimmed hat with a huge ostrich feather and my quiet unassuming husband was a dashing cavalier. I think he quite enjoyed the role. The only problem was, whenever he lit a cigar, the ostrich feather nearly went up in smoke.

As we left home, we felt a right pair of 'charlies'. However, when we got to the Tithebarn, we found that by comparison with some of the other guests' outfits, we looked positively plain. One lot came as The Flintstones and on arrival presented their 'card' – a piece of rock with their names scratched on it.

Another chap had cut up his wife's fur coat to come as a cave man and an Elizabethan gentleman in short cape, doublet and hose, headed in the direction of the loo with an anxious expression, muttering: 'I don't know how the hell I'm going to manage this!' As his short 16th-century style pants were padded out to the required shape with toilet rolls, we didn't think he'd have too many problems.

John, our host, was the court jester, dressed in red and yellow pointed tunic, with a bell at the end of each point and also on his hat and slippers. Brenda was a 1920s flapper.

The assembled company left their inhibitions at the door, along with their coats. Observations and comments on the various outfits prompted wit and laughter and a jovial atmosphere. Seating was supplemented with bales of straw, we ate our fill and sang all the old songs, e.g. 'Down at the old Bull and Bush', etc. from song sheets John had provided. Several soloists sang or recited, adding to the homemade entertainment. It also added another four-figure sum to the Fund and my dashing cavalier couldn't remember when he'd last enjoyed himself so much.

The world of Sport has made a fine contribution to the Fund. At Sir William Downward's invitation, Sir Matt Busby, Chairman of Manchester United Football Club and one of the most respected men in the game, had agreed to be a Patron of the Fund. Supporters' Clubs held fund-raising events and football stars made appearances at functions or attended them to receive cheques on behalf of the Fund. Practically every north-west club in the FA made some contribution. Many clubs donated autographed footballs, some clubs donated players' fines incurred during the season and we even had a ball signed by the England team. On Boxing Day, local Lions Clubs provided a group of volunteers under the leadership of Garstang Lions President, Jim Vale. They came to help with a collection at Preston North End's ground, for which the Football League had granted permission. The collection outside the ground was done with our collecting tins which proved to be a harmless exercise when compared with the one inside the ground during the half-time interval. This was done with blankets, into which the crowd threw coins. Before they began, I said a few words on the public address system.

Geoff took part in this and afterwards said that he wished he'd had a crash helmet. He had quite a few lumps on his head, and Lion Brian Prentice collected quite a nasty gash. Some people's aim wasn't very good and the men just hoped that their bruises were caused by 50p pieces and not 10p pieces! However, it raised several hundred pounds.

After Boxing Day, I took a week off the 'Scanner Trail'. For those few days, I was just 'Mum', enjoying the time with my family, doing my share of the cooking and the washing up, visiting friends I'd neglected or just spending the evenings watching the television or reading a book – the latter being a rare luxury.

Talking of books, Mike had bought me *The Frank Muir Book: an Irreverent Companion to Social History* for Christmas. Under the section entitled Literature, Frank describes the writer Harriet Martineau as a 'woman with a frail hold on life who got through enough work to cripple a carthorse'.

I knew just how she must have felt. But I wondered if she had found her work half so rewarding, or so heartwarming, as I found my self-appointed task?

7

The Trail Branches

By New Year's Day, 1978 there were fifty branches of the Appeal Fund, in various places in the north-west.

What sort of people are they, these men and women who have volunteered to help me?

They come from all walks of life, from all strata of society. They include the affluent and those of limited resources. They are professional people, trades people, business people, factory workers and housewives. All that mattered to me was that their hearts should be in the right place; that they should be honest and reliable. Many of them are, like me, patients of the Christie, who are still receiving treatment. Others are former patients who are now cured; still more are those who have lost relatives, or who have relatives who have cancer. Some see helping the Fund as a matter of social responsibility.

Whatever their reasons for helping, all of these men and women have put in hours and hours of work on a voluntary basis. They had held their own fund-raising functions. They have attended events in support of the Fund which have been arranged by other groups and organisations in their areas. They have received cheques and thanked the donors on behalf of the Fund. Their contribution to the success of the Appeal has been invaluable.

By the end of 1977 I had met quite a lot of these men and women but many were still only known to me as voices on the telephone or through their letters. When the Fund became a registered charity, former letters of authority were withdrawn. New letters, typed on my official stationery and which stated the charity number, were issued. These letters were signed by me and give the names of the officials of the branch; the chairman, secretary and treasurer. The original letter is retained by the chairman and photocopies are given to each member of the committee.

In pursuit of personal interests and as a journalist, I have seen a great deal of committee work. My recommendation to the branches was to keep their committees *small*. Large committees are cumbersome. They can lead to friction and to a great deal of waffling, with no decisions being reached. There can be clashes of personality and a lowering of morale, for invariably, there is always one individual on large committees – not necessarily the chairman – who tries to assume the role of dictator and takes every opinion at variance with his own as a personal affront. Therefore, I recommended that six people were sufficient, for it is far better to have half a dozen people who can work together harmoniously and constructively than to spend most of the time holding committee meetings at which the main purpose seems to be to placate abrasive factions. It is also an advantage to have an outer periphery of friends who will help out when the occasion warrants it. Some people are perfectly willing to assist at odd events, whereas they may not have the time, or the inclinations to help on a regular basis.

Another fact which I have tried to get across is that there are no 'bosses' on this Appeal. I am the founder and the Appeal is in my name. As such, I am 'the front man', here to give advice if it is asked for, to make recommendations and to help in any way I can, but the emphasis is on teamwork. We are all part of the team, including the medical and the lay people on the Central Committee.

There are no strict territorial boundaries. It is preferable that there should not be jealously guarded demarcation lines between once branch and another. For example, let's take two adjacent branches: a committee member of Branch A may have a friend who lives within Branch B's area and who wishes to help her by putting on a fund-raising effort. In this case, it is courteous if Branch A would mention it to Branch B.

Branch B's attitude should be 'fine – go ahead' for it really doesn't matter which branch treasurer pays in the money. We are all working for the same Fund. Similarly, if a group or organisation in Branch A's area asks for a representative to attend their meeting, either to talk about the Appeal or to be presented with a cheque – and none of Branch A's committee are able to go on that date in question, it is helpful if they have established a sufficiently good relationship to be able to ring members of Branch B's committee to see if they can take on the engagement.

There need be no competition between branches; the accent is on co-operation, co-operation all along the line. Competition is negative. It is a complete waste of time and effort and can create unnecessary ill will.

We arranged to have a meeting of the branches and asked that each committee send their delegate to the Christie on Saturday, 21st January. Of the fifty branches, thirty-seven were represented, but even as the invitations went out, I knew that one person would not be there.

Mrs Flo' Wilson of Prestbury had been a tireless worker for the Fund. In a few short months she had raised several hundred pounds. We had some lively telephone conversations and she wrote some amusing letters to me. They were full of information about her fund-raising activities. Sometimes they were almost illegible because she didn't even have time to change the ribbon on her typewriter.

Just before Christmas, Flo' had written to tell me she would be off the road for a while and wouldn't be able to attend the branch meeting. She said she was going into hospital for an operation immediately after Christmas, but after a suitable period of convalescence, she would resume her fund-raising activities. On the second day of the New Year, Flo's husband telephoned to tell me that his wife had died – of cancer. It was a bitter blow for him. He said that he took comfort in the fact that Flo' had died in the same way that she had lived – quickly and without fuss.

Flo' and I had never met, but through our letters and our telephone conversations, she was the kind of woman I knew I would instinctively like, when I did meet her. I felt as though I had lost a friend.

At the branch meeting, it was good to meet people and to be able to put faces to the names I knew so well.

I began by introducing the members of the Central Committee, my husband Geoff (to whom many had spoken on the phone), and also introduced Mr Ron Walker, Liaison Officer of the Fund and his wife, Sylvia. Then, Sir William chaired the meeting.

EMI's film *The Scanner Story* was screened. It effectively shows the potential of Computerised Axial Tomography. One sequence shows the scanners being crated for shipment to hospitals in many parts of the world – over 1,000 of them. When the film was made in 1976, the total in British hospitals hardly reached double figures. It recharged our enthusiasm to make sure that the Christie got theirs!

Dr Eddleston then spoke about the hospital's need of CAT; how it would benefit patients and how it would make the diagnosis of the disease and the planning of treatment easier and more accurate, and with a resultant saving of life.

For some time, I had been concerned that I might lose otherwise willing helpers because they could no longer afford to do the work. I knew full well that there is a limit to how many stamps one can buy, how many telephone calls one can make, how much petrol one can put in the tank of one's car and keep standing the cost out of one's own pocket.

The Fund Treasurer, Mr Geoffrey Ball, gave some advice on simple accounting procedures, showing how the expenses incurred in putting on an event should be deducted from the profits of that event and the balance paid into the main fund account. Duplicated sheets, showing several examples of how accounts should be kept, were circulated. As each new branch has been formed, a copy has been sent to its treasurer.

We then adjourned for lunch, after which Mr Calderwood explained to delegates some of the legal aspects of the Appeal; what the law allows one to do and also some of the pitfalls to be avoided.

Mr Douglas Emmett, editor of the *Manchester Evening News*, and I then spoke about publicity; how to seek the co-operation of local newspapers. It's not a bit of good ringing a local newspaper in the morning to tell them that you are holding some kind of function that evening. On a weekly paper, the diary for the following week is usually arranged on the day of publication. A photographer may have six or more jobs to cover in one evening. He and the sub-editors will arrange which of them will take precedence, for it may well be a physical impossibility for him to get round all of them. Then there is always the unexpected occurrence. For example: say there is your coffee evening, a presentation being made by the Mayor and two or three other events; it could be that your coffee evening is missed out so that the Mayor's presentation is covered. On the other hand, if a local factory goes up in smoke that night, then the Mayor may have 'had it' as well. But the more notice one can give, the better the chances of a photographer and reporter turning up. Local news reportage of events are important to a charity. People reading about what has taken place may very well be encouraged to do something to help and in this way, the support grows and gathers pace.

Julé Hayward was then asked to tell members about her brilliant fund-raising idea, but that is a chapter in itself . . .

The afternoon ended with a general discussion and a question-and-answer session. We all went home feeling that the meeting had been useful and constructive. What is more, most of us went home feeling we'd made a whole lot of new friends. We could now put faces and personalities to the names on the list of branches.

During 1978 more branches were formed. For various reasons, such as moving away from the district, or illness, branches in some areas ceased to exist. Others took their place and by the end of the year there were ·sixty-eight branches. Their enthusiasm, their hard work and the ideas they came up with had to be seen to be believed. Because of the Appeal and the many people who have seen fit to help, Geoff and I now have a much wider circle of friends. We have spent many evenings with members of the branch committees, attending functions. Nice people, good people . . . we count ourselves all the richer for knowing them.

Geoff cannot always come with me on my travels. As he puts it, 'someone has to keep the house door open', and he does have his own commitments. But whenever possible he accompanies me and I'm always glad when he does, for we have few evenings at home together. As a result we have friends in many parts of the north-west. They are friendships which will probably continue long after the Appeal has reached its objective. Branch committee members tell me the same thing. Through working for the Appeal, they have been to many places and met many people they would not other-wise have known. Like me, they have been amazed and inspired by the many acts of kindness, by the goodwill and the examples of outstanding generosity. My branch committee know exactly what I mean when I refer to what has taken place as 'The North-West Miracle'. They've witnessed so much of it themselves. To the sceptic, I would say that had you taken part, had you trodden the 'Scanner Trail' with us, you would know beyond all doubt that the age of miracles is not yet past.

On many occasions I have spent a full day in a north-west town – places such as Wigan, Bolton or a district of the City of Manchester. The object has been that I spend the day trying to meet as many as possible of the people in that area who have helped.

For example, we have three branches in the Bolton area and four in the Wigan area. The day's itinerary is arranged by the branch committees, for they know their area better than I. They know which factory, which school or college, which individuals would appreciate a visit from me. We pack into the day as much as is humanly possible. Reaching the town at about 10 a.m. it has sometimes been close to midnight when I have driven home along the motorway. A typical day in Bolton included visits to three factories, two primary schools, two secondary schools, Bolton Technical College, followed in the evening by a visit to a fashion show at one venue and a dance at another – all in support of the Fund.

Such days can be physically exhausting, but they have given me the opportunity to meet and thank at least *some* of the many people who have contributed. Wherever I have gone, I have been received with warmth and affection. This is something I could not have foreseen. I hope that those I met know that their help is appreciated and not taken for granted. The Appeal may have started as a personal venture on my part, but a vast army of people of goodwill have taken it to their hearts and we are all in it together. I like to think that such visits helped to unite us, so that we could identify with each other and with the cause for which we are all working. Another aspect of these visits is that I have seen manufacturing procedures in factories I would have had no occasion to visit, but for the Appeal. I have found them of great interest and as a result, many of the commodities I have watched being produced, now remind me of the people I have met whose job it is to make them.

For example, have you ever wondered how that tight paper seal inside a tin of custard powder is affixed so neatly? No? Neither had I until I saw how it was done. Visiting Metal Box Company's Clayton factory with Mrs Edith Jones, chairman of the North Manchester branch, I watched with rapt attention as the automated assembly line converted carboard and metal into drum-shaped containers, complete with a well-known brand-name label. They would be sent to the custard powder firm like this, where they would be filled and the base affixed. It sounds an upside-down process – which it is – but when you think about it, it's common sense. The same procedure is used for other commodities, such as scouring powders, etc. This firm made the Appeal's collecting boxes.

With Mrs Jean Wootton, chairman of the Bury Metropolitan branch, I visited Cusson's soap factory at Kersall. We watched several well-known brands of soap being produced. From huge vats, and like toothpaste coming out of an outsize tube, there emerged gigantic ribbons of hot pliable soap, cooling as it progressed along the production line. In various stages, it is cut, shaped, stamped with the brand name and wrapped. Then each dozen or so tablets of soap are polythene sealed by automatic process, ready for packing into cardboard boxes. At this final stage, the soap is still warm, but by the time it reaches the shops it is cold, hard and firm. I was given four tablets of their luxury soap, a brand we don't see in Britain as it's for export only.

Having washed and ironed endless pairs of my son's and

daughter's denim jeans over the years, I was extremely interested to visit Courtauld's spinning mill at Coppull. Here, the thread which will eventually be woven into hard-wearing denim fabric is produced and it is in this factory that Mrs Marian Davies, a Christie patient and a member of the Higher Ince committee, works. The raw Colombian cotton arrives at the mill full of impurities. It is cleaned, carded and combed and blended with polyester man-made fibre – seventy per cent cotton to thirty per cent polyester. It emerges from the machines as a long soft skein, rather like cotton wool and about three fingers thick. It then gets its first spinning, the skein being stretched to seven times its length and twisted to what seems like thick string and wound on to a 'cop'. Then comes a further spinning. The 'thick string' is twisted and spun to twelve times its length and wound onto more 'cops'. It is now similar in appearance to a forties crochet cotton and at this stage has the required strength, durability and elasticity. Some is wound on to what look like outsize versions of the ordinary domestic cotton reels, hundreds of threads on one reel, which weavers at another factory will use as the warp of the fabric. Thread on 'cops' and subsequently on flying shuttles, will form the weft. Thus the fabric is produced. It will be dyed, sent to cutters and machinists before it arrives on shop counters or market stalls as denim jeans or skirts or jackets. It was extremely interesting and I brought home some samples of the cotton and polyester at the various stages, for the children of one of our local schools. The educational budget allows little spare money for schools to make such visits. I brought the school more samples from Darwen when I saw another manufacturing process at Crown Wallpaper Company's Potter's Mill.

The employees had a Sick Club Fund for many decades, but recently the firm provided a similar facility. The workers had elected that the money in the now defunct Sick Club should go to the Fund, rather than be shared out among them. On the day they presented Mrs Lilian Scott, chairman of the Darwen Branch, and myself with a cheque I was taken on a tour of the factory. They have a strike here, every week – only it's no industrial dispute! In fact they haven't had one at this factory since the turn of the century, which is a fine record. But then, there's a happy family atmosphere at Potter's Mill and some employees have put in thirty or forty years of service. 'Strike' is their word for when a new pattern goes on the printing machines.

Ever wondered how vinyl wallpapers are coated? Never having given the matter much thought, I think I would have guessed that this is the last part of the process. I'd have been quite wrong – it's the first. The huge rolls of paper – 63 inches wide – are unrolled and conveyed over a vat, where they are sprayed with liquid vinyl. Proceeding through a drying compartment, they are re-rolled. The rolls are then machine cut into 21-inch standard wallpaper width. Then the pattern is struck, machines printing it in five stages. Sections of pattern and colour are superimposed progressively until the design is completed, then heat treatment fuses the pattern and vinyl together. More machines roll and cut the paper into the standard 33-feet lengths; they are labelled, put into polythene tubes which are heat shrunk to provide tight, protective seals and are now ready for distribution. We also saw the pattern books being made, from which customers would make their selection and in the design room, we watched the artists at work. Here was the amateur watching the professionals . . . it was enough to make me give up painting altogether! I know that whenever I next buy wallpaper, I will think of those nice friendly folk I met at Potter's Mill and wonder if any of them had a hand in its making.

There have been many other factories, some of whose assembly line procedures have absolutely baffled me. A visit to the Lucas Switchgear factory at Burnley is a case in point.

When Julé Hayward and I visited it, I watched ladies assembling unidentifiable components, handling the minutest bits and pieces with an unbelievable speed and dexterity. I'd like to have had a go, but I know I'd suddenly have found that I had ten thumbs! However, there was no doubt about the warmth of the welcome. The girls had done a great deal to help the Fund. They are a jolly crowd of Lancashire lasses, genuine, full of good humour and typical northern generosity.

Another fascinating and equally mysterious assembly line – but on a more gigantic scale – came within my orbit during a visit to the British Aerospace factory in Manchester. Everyone knew exactly what they were doing, down to the last thousandth of an inch. The results were huge aircraft fuselages, and wings, but yours truly was more at home in the canteen, drinking coffee and having a chat with the staff and some of those employed on the production floor. Come to think of it, I suppose the skills involved in the production of a newspaper and watching it go to press, are interesting when you haven't seen it before. I know that I have found it very interesting indeed to have seen how some of the commodities I had previously taken for granted are produced. I have a new appreciation of the work and planning that goes into them before they reach the public. Even more, I've enjoyed meeting the people who make them. But then, as Geoff is so fond of telling folk – especially if we are in a district new to us – 'If it's a choice between a tour of the vicinity to admire the scenery, or spending the time meeting and talking to people, Pat will plump for people every time.'

If we had branches of the Fund in various places throughout the north-west, we had one – or as good as one – at the very centre of things. I refer to the administration staff of the Christie. Over the months, David Critchley the Hospital Sector Administrator and I had become good friends. We had argued, fought and compromised and evolved a mutual respect for each other. When David, in search of promotion, left the Christie to take up another post in the Midlands, I wasn't the only one who viewed his departure with regret. David's right hand in the Christie, was Susan Dawson, his secretary and she now fulfils that role for David's successor. Together with her assistant, Pam Barber, they run an extremely busy office, working at full stretch, answering calls on any one of four telephones coming from inside or outside the hospital; dealing with queries from all departments of the hospital, be it a doctor asking that arrangements be made for a symposium or the catering staff asking for extra help.

I have been in that office many times when it was impossible to get a word in edgeways, for people coming through the door, firing questions, in the middle of which one of the phones would ring . . . before either Susan or Pam had finished answering it, someone else would come in, seeking information about another matter.

The Appeal has placed an extra workload on that office. There have been periods, after national publicity of one kind or another, when they have had over a hundred extra letters in addition to the average daily amount of mail which in itself is formidable. How these two girls have coped with it, is beyond me, but they have done so, cheerfully and without complaint, putting in hours of extra time on behalf of the Fund, far and away beyond the boundaries of their normal work. Whatever I have asked of them, they have always managed to come up with the answer, or fit in yet one more extra job.

Susan says, 'Some nights, we go home with our brains addled and feeling utterly exhausted. But we identify with the Appeal – it's our contribution.'

The same goes for other members of the Christie staff. Doctors have attended meetings of interested organisations to talk about the Appeal or to receive donations; the girls on the reception desk in Outpatients Department have had a collecting box on the desk, held raffles, sold our pens and our badges; the WRVS ladies who provide cups of tea in that Department have held their own fund-raising efforts and brought the money into the hospital . . . and so it goes – inside as well as outside the Christie, everyone was doing all that they could, to help.

If the Christie administration liaised with the Branches at their end, Ron Walker became my 'long stop' at the Garstang end. Like me, Ron was born in Salford. In his younger days he'd been a Rugby League player for the Salford RFC. He and his wife and daughter now live in Garstang and I had first met Ron at Garstang Town Council meetings. He as a councillor and I as a reporter.

Shortly after the Fund was launched, Ron had called to see me. He had written to Mr Brian Snape, the chairman of Salford Rugby Club and the Willows Leisure and Variety Centre. As a result, he became involved in organising a charity night at the club and later, arranged several similar functions at night clubs and other venues up and down the north-west.

When I ran out of steam, Ron took over. If I was out on the 'Scanner Trail' and one of the branch committees wanted information, they knew they could ring Ron and more than likely, he'd be able to tell them what they wanted to know. If some unexpected 'date' presented itself and I was due to go somewhere else, I could rely on Ron to fulfil the date for me, at short notice. In spite of a reputed toughness on the rugby field, Ron is as kindly and good-natured a man as you could meet. He and his wife Sylvia have been extremely loyal to Geoff and me and staunch supporters of the Fund. My 'long stop' became our close friend.

Each of the branch committees could probably fill a book with their own account of things which have happened to them in the course of working for the Appeal. Like myself, they have faced and coped with some tragic situations and equally, they have had their hilarious moments. One chairman attended a charity night and on the bill was a snake charmer. As the person representing the Appeal she was a 'natural' target and when the charmer came down among the audience, the poor girl ended up having a 12-foot boa constrictor wrapped around her neck. She all but passed out! A night to remember? She's not likely to forget it!

Another member received a phone call which resulted in a visit which ended in some embarrassment. I write it, just as it was told to me, via the telephone, on her return home.

This took place in a country district. My representative's phone rang. She picked it up and gave her number, to which a voice replied.

'About that there Fund . . .'

'Oh yes?'

'I'd like to give summat to it.'

'That's very kind of you. Do you want to send it directly to Pat or the Christie, or would you like me to come to see you?'

'Tha' can come and see me – and tha'd better come between four and five.'

'Oh. Yes. That will be all right. I'll come to see you this afternoon.'

Just after four o'clock, my branch member arrived at an old-fashioned farmhouse. She was shown into the kitchen, which had a black Yorkshire range, with a high mantel-shelf, cluttered with ornaments in the centre of which was a photograph of a man. In one corner of the kitchen was a large old-fashioned slop stone sink, circa 1890.

'Sit thee down, lass,' invited the elderly farmer's wife. She turfed the cat off an old horsehair sofa to provide a seat for my friend and for a while they exchanged polite conversation. Eventually, the mistress of the house produced her purse and took out some notes. As she handed her donation over she did so with a nod in the direction of the picture on the mantel-piece and with the words: 'Only I thought as how Ah'd better ask thee to come whilst *he* was out. Tha' knows, he pees in t'sink!'

The branch member made some non-committal remark and made her escape just as soon as she could.

The Wigan Branch of the Fund appeared on television as the jury in the Granada programme 'Crown Court'. They paid their remuneration into the Fund. And the chairman of one branch of the Appeal, who is a mastectomy patient, defied the local press to tell which of her breasts was her own and which was a bag of bird seed!

There is no doubt that the 'Scanner Trail' has provided a whole lot of new experiences for us all!

8

'A Bloody Good Idea'

One day in November 1977, Julé Hayward phoned. After exchanging pleasantries and enquiring about each other's health, she said:

'Pat, do you remember that very first telephone conversation we had? If you remember, you said that all that was needed were a million people who would each give 75p – and that would be it. We'd be home and dry. Well, I've had an idea and I think it could work.'

'No, I don't remember . . . wait a minute . . . yes, I do. Why? What have you got in mind?'

'You know this craze for wearing badges?'

'Yes.'

'Everybody wears badges of one kind or another these days. Young people, especially, like them. They wear them plastered all over their anoraks or coats. Even adults wear certain badges. How would it be if we had a million badges made to sell at 50p? The Fund is almost at the quarter of a million mark now. This could bring in the other half million we need.'

'It could be a good idea,' I said cautiously, thinking of the possibilities. 'It would need promoting properly, with plenty of publicity . . . What would you have on the badge?'

'If we had a million people all supporting the Fund, they'd all be one in a million, wouldn't they? How about "I'm One in a Million"?'

'They would have to include some reference to the Fund as well, so that people knew what they were buying them for. How are you going to get all that on a small badge?'

'I know someone who will draw some designs for us. I'll ask him to let me have a few alternative drawings, then we'll have an idea what will be best. The badges wouldn't have to be big, or no one would wear them. Something about the size of a 10p piece would be about right, I should think,' said Julé.

'Do you think it's a bit much to ask 50p for a small badge?'

'No. I don't. We wouldn't pretend that a badge was actually worth 50p. It's a way of making a 50p donation – and by wearing it, being seen to support the Fund.'

'There's one other thing we've got to think about, Julé. A lot will depend on how much it's going to cost to have the badges made. Have you had any thoughts on that?'

She laughed.

'I know we have pleaded, cajoled and even bullied lots of folk into doing things for nothing for the Fund, but I don't think we could ask any firm to produce a million badges free of charge.'

'I know. Somebody told me the other day that I could sell ice to the Eskimos. I was twisting his arm about something and ended up paying half the proper price, bless him . . . but we couldn't ask for something on *that* scale for free.'

'Paddy and I will make some enquiries. I'll give you a ring when I've something to report.'

Julé's enthusiasm was infectious. What is more, she was an educational psychologist before her marriage. Since she'd offered to help me in July, she and her husband, Patrick, a director of a Rossendale firm of dyers, had rallied support in

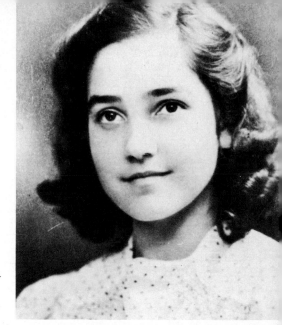

Pat Seed at fourteen
(Pat Seed)

The Lancashire lad and lass.
With Russell Harty – who
was not such an ogre after
all (London Weekend
Television)

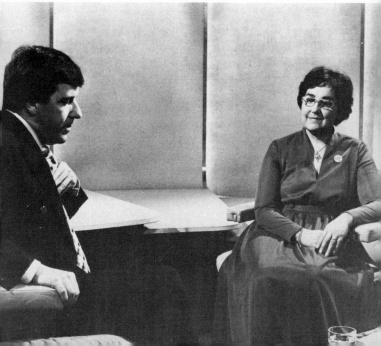

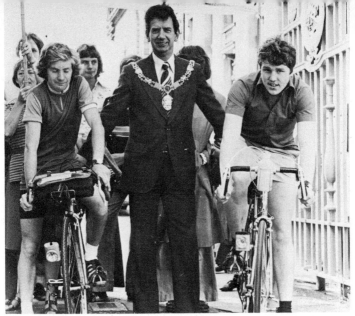

The start of a sponsored cycle ride from Lancaster to Land's End by two 16-year-old boys, Steven Parkinson and David Tuer, sent on their way by the Mayor of Lancaster, Councillor Harry Holgate *(Lancaster Guardian)*

With two-year-old cancer patient Clair and her mother at Chorley *(Chorley Guardian)*

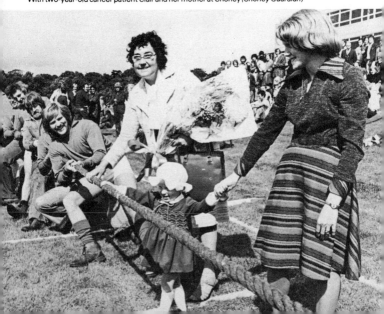

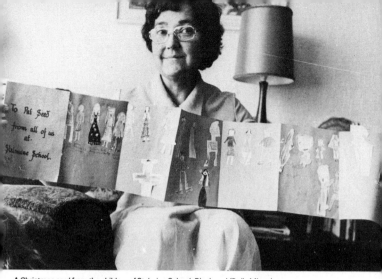

A Christmas card from the children of Stalmine School, Blackpool *(Daily Mirror)*

Terry Arnold walks the Pennine Way – in a week! *(Stockport Express)*

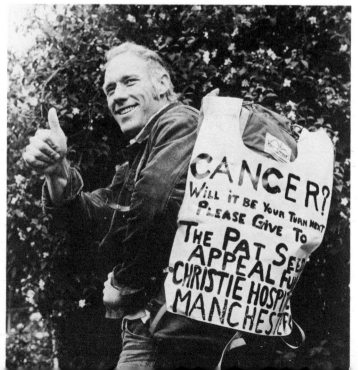

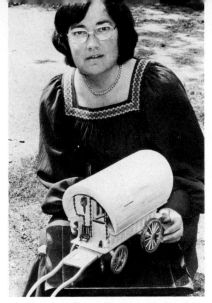

A gypsy caravan made of matchsticks for the fund by Richard, a prisoner *(Daily Express)*

With Red Rum and Mrs Beryl McCain who is presenting a cheque from the stables
(Lancashire Evening Post)

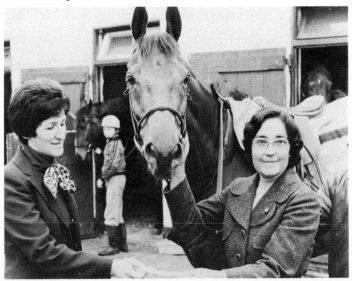

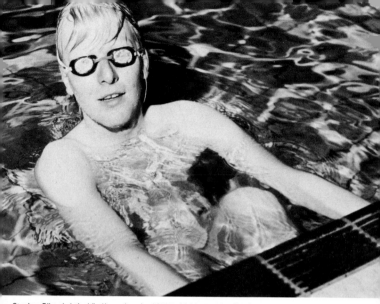

Stephen Bilynskyj, the blind boy who raised £700 with his sponsored swim
(Oldham Evening Chronicle)

The kids who made it a million! Children of Northfold County Infants School, Cleveleys, whose cheque took the fund over the £1 million mark *(Daily Express)*

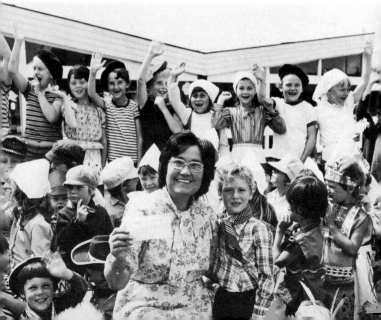

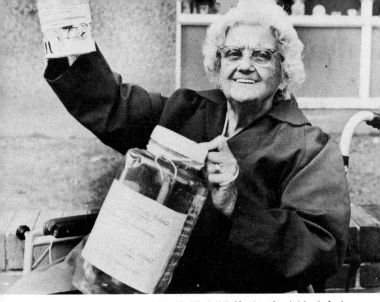

Being confined to a wheelchair doesn't deter Mrs Minnie Hall of Stockport from helping the fund
(Manchester Evening News)

12 October 1977, the night Ken Dodd became a patron of the fund: *left to right* Ken Dodd, Pat Seed,
Robert Dickinson, treasurer of the South Ribble branch (County Photographic Services Stockport Ltd)

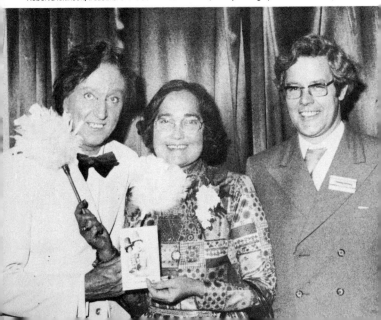

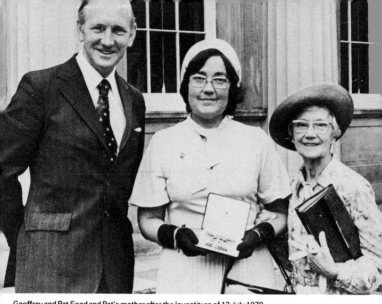

Geoffrey and Pat Seed and Pat's mother after the Investiture of 12 July 1978
(United Newspapers Ltd London)

Mrs Snowdon, Pat Seed, Dr Hounsfield and Nicola Farrow make sure that the stone is well and truly
laid *(West Lancs Evening Gazette)*

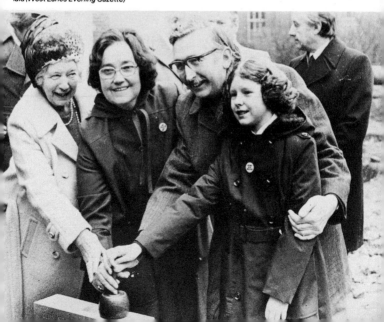

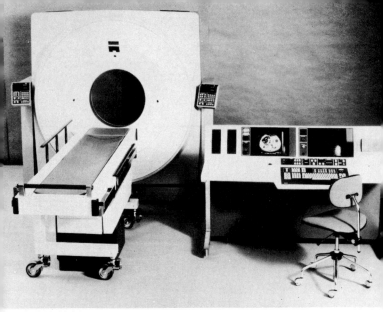

The EMI Scanner 7070 and control panel (EMI Medical Ltd)
A patient being put into position for CT diagnosis (EMI Medical Ltd)

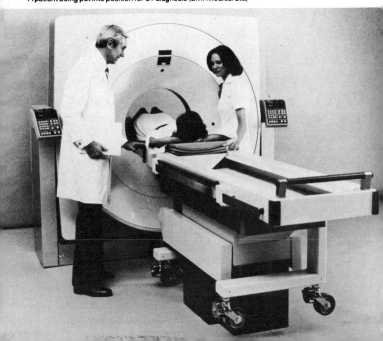

the Burnley, Nelson and Colne areas, getting plenty of coverage in the local newspapers. (*Whatever you are doing, let your local papers know!*) Journalists on local papers had given excellent coverage and every possible help. They'd done a fine job and made a valuable contribution.

So had Julé. Possessing a charming personality and full of ideas, she had thought up all kinds of money-raising schemes and put them into practice. A mastectomy patient and far from well, I know that on many occasions she had dragged herself out of bed, put her best face on and her best foot forward and attended some event to receive a donation and say a few words of thanks – and then gone home and crawled back into bed again. Sometimes, our telephone conversations would be via our bedside phones. We'd each ask how the other was feeling, have a good moan to each other and then try to boost each other's morale. For us both, the philosophy was the same – one day at a time.

Some days later, Julé rang again.

'We've got some designs. The one Paddy and I like best is "I'm One in a Million" in black lettering on a yellow background. In dotted lettering behind the words, is the name Pat Seed.'

'Can't you get "Appeal Fund" on it? It will look big headed – as though *I'm* one in a million.'

'No. To get all that on a badge of this size, you'd hardly be able to read any of it.'

'I'd be happier if it mentioned the Fund. That's what's important, not me.'

'I think you'll be satisfied when you see them,' said Julé.

'Now for the crucial question – do we know what it's going to cost?'

'Yes, we do. Are you sitting down?'

'Yes . . . is it as bad as all that?'

'Hold your breath – about £18,000 to £20,000!'

'Oh my stars! That puts it right out of the question!'

145

The Fund was gathering pace. The rate the money was coming in was accelerating more quickly than I could have hoped for in my wildest dreams. But we hadn't had it long enough to cover an outlay of this magnitude out of the interest, especially when interest rates had taken a tumble and almost halved during 1977. Not only was I determined that there should be no capital withdrawals for whatever reason, I was doing everything possible to maintain our slogan 'Every donation one hundred per cent for the Scanner'. As I said earlier, I was tired of charities where a large percentage of the money donated went in high administrative costs before the residue found its way to the cause for which it had been given. That was not for me or for a Fund which bore my name. I just could not speculate with Fund money, much of which was widows' mites or children's pocket money. I was pretty sure the Central Committee would take the same view.

I said as much to Julé.

'It's a brilliant scheme, love, and it could very well work, even though a million badges would take an awful lot of shifting. I daresay the branches would sell them and other people would, too, but we just can't speculate with £18,000 to £20,000.'

A few days later Julé rang again and provided the answer.

She and Paddy had such faith in their idea, they agreed to put up the money. They were prepared to take the risk.

'Are you absolutely sure this is what you want to do? It's a splendid offer, Julé, and it leaves me speechless. I don't know what your financial resources are, but it's a heck of a lot of money to lose if it doesn't pay off.'

'I know it is. I could have nightmares about it if I didn't keep a hold on myself!' she giggled.

'Nightmares! I wouldn't even sleep!'

'Oh, come on, Pat – what's money? You and I both know there are more important things in life than that!'

'Julé, it's a marvellous offer. Are you perfectly certain that

146

this is what you want to do? Hadn't you better think about it a bit more?'

'No. We've made up our minds. Paddy and I have discussed it and we're prepared to take the chance.'

'I don't know how to even begin to say thank you. But one thing is certain – whatever the bill comes to, the first money to come in from the sale of the badges will be yours. You'll be reimbursed at the first possible moment.'

'Publicity is going to be all important. Paddy thought of having a few larger, non-reflective badges made for press purposes.'

'It's not only going to be important, Julé, it's going to be vital. Leave that one with me. We'll bring it up at the branch meeting in January and see what the delegates think about it. A lot is going to depend on them.'

And so we did.

A couple of days before the meeting, Julé had gone into hospital again for yet more treatment, but her doctors had agreed to let her out for the day so that she could be with us. In the interim, Julé and I had more discussions, getting down to the practicalities. It would be towards the end of February before the manufacturers could supply the first batch. Allowing for possible late delivery, plus the distribution to branches in all parts of the north-west, we decided to launch the scheme on 1st March. I said I would send a press-release to all north-west provincial newspapers and the national dailies, plus a copy to all branches of the Fund. We would ask each branch to present the first badge in their area to the Mayor of their town, borough or city, making sure that the arrangements were convenient to the local paper as well as to the mayor.

When the delegates at the branch meeting heard of the scheme, I think the first reaction was one of awe that the Haywards were prepared to risk so much money. However, they were quick to realise the scheme's possibilities and that much of its success would depend on them.

'You are not expected to sell every single badge yourselves. You couldn't possibly do it. You all know your own areas. Get them into every office, shop or factory where you know someone who is willing to sell them,' I said. 'Just as I rely on you to help me, so you must rely on other people to help you sell the badges.'

Delegate, delegate . . . it was vital if the scheme was to succeed. The sooner Paddy and Julé were reimbursed, the happier I'd be.

The Nat-West opened a special account for the badge scheme and every branch treasurer had a special paying-in book. When the badges were launched on the first day of March, the Fund total was nearing the half million mark. But by then had come the realisation that our original target figure of three quarters of a million wasn't going to be enough. Estimates drawn up by the Christie staff in 1976 were now way out of date. How much did we need? At this point, no one could say for certain. It could be well over a million pounds. Not only had the whole scheme been hit by inflation, technology was progressing. The 'second generation' scanners were faster, with better imagery. They were also more expensive. The bitterest blow of all was to learn that staffing costs would have to include the salaries and wages of everyone employed in the new department, even those of the domestic cleaners, whereas the original figure had estimated the salaries of a couple of radiographers.

What it boiled down to was a cold, hard fact. The government would not give *one single penny*. It was disheartening and depressing.

The technical people on the central committee went away to do their homework and that was no simple bit of arithmetic either; no pat, ready answer, but involving round after round of enquiries, discussions and consultations. Far from making us throw in the towel, it renewed our determination yet again. OK – so we needed more money. How much, we did not know. We could only hazard a guess. But we would get that scanner at the Christie, or BUST! Meanwhile, Paddy and half a dozen of his friends drove in all directions, all over the north-west, delivering boxes of badges.

Quiet and unassuming, Paddy was like an army general, directing operations and supplying the troops in the field with ammunition. The badges were signed for right along the line, by the branch committees and by the people to whom they delegated them. On special forms, we have an account of exactly who has had how many and where.

My printer, Colin, worked overtime to produce thousands of posters, black lettering on a yellow paper to match the badges. Our sorting office coped with yet another batch of sixty-odd parcels, for the number of branches was ever increasing. Some of the posters were worded: 'Are You "One in a Million"?', and others: 'Give 50p and be "One in a Million".'

Practically every north-west newspaper carried the story, together with a picture of a Mayor being presented with a badge by members of the local committee.

A news editor on the *Lancashire Evening Post* said: 'Pat, we'll help you all we can, but there's a limit to the number of pictures of mayors wearing badges we can use. We've printed four or five already.' I realised that. The circulation area stretches from Kendal to Chorley (north to south) and to points east and west. There's an awful lot of mayors in a territory that size and the *Post* had certainly given me a fair crack of the whip. As well as newspaper coverage, broadcasts on several local radio stations also helped things along. In Burnley, Julé's young son and daughter presented a badge to the Mayor of Pendle. Mummy was back in hospital again.

One morning I received a letter from Jean Wootton, chairman of the Bury Metro Branch. Jean said that she had not been able to sleep the night before and had come downstairs to make herself a cup of tea. Sitting there in the quiet of her kitchen, an idea had come to her and she reached for a pencil. Several cups of tea later, the result was a poem, a copy of which she enclosed. It was good in that it explained to those who had heard of neither the Appeal nor the badge scheme, just what the whole thing was about. I rang Jean to ask if she'd any objection to my using her poem. She hadn't, and Colin printed it and we distributed the posters far and wide.

> Are you that one in a million?
> Are you that face in a crowd?
> Are you wearing one of our badges?
> If you are, then you can be proud.
> For you're helping to buy the CAT Scanner
> Which the Christie so desperately need.
> You're fulfilling the dream of a Northern lass,
> The woman you know as Pat Seed.
> Thank you for buying our badges,
> Your 50p will unlock the doors.
> We will fight this battle called cancer
> Remember –
> THE LIFE YOU HELP SAVE COULD BE YOURS!
>
> Jean Wootton,
> Chairman, Bury Metropolitan Branch

The badge idea was Julé's, the poem was Jean's; we were all selling them wherever we could, making use of every outlet we could think of. Soroptimists through the north-west sold them, Women's Institutes sold them. Ladies Circles sold them and on Garstang market, Circlers sold them on a market stall for three successive Thursdays. Journalists and front office staff of national and provincial newspapers sold them, including those of the *Salford City Reporter*, the paper that had printed my first journalistic efforts. At the *Gazette* in Blackpool, Pat Hunter sold nearly four thousand pounds worth of them. Readers had also sent in books of trading stamps which added £4,000 to the Fund, via Sue Naylor, chairman of the Fleetwood Branch. Staff of National Dailies – the *Express*, the *Mail*, the *Mirror* and the *Telegraph* – also sold badges.

For someone whose formative years had included the Manchester and Salford blitz, this was a blitzkrieg of a different kind and it was loaded with goodwill. We bombarded the north-west with badges and they captured the imagination of the public as the Appeal itself was doing. In addition, many branch members sent them to relatives in other parts of the country and several batches went overseas. Through various contacts, they were sold on the Manchester and the London Stock Exchanges. In the House of Commons, they became the insignia of every north-west Member of Parliament. Suddenly, it seemed that at all points of the compass there were people sporting our bright yellow badges, all proud to be 'One in a Million'. It became the 'in' thing. If you hadn't a badge, you weren't 'with it'. And as the badges were sold, the stories about them came in thick and fast . . .

At a nightclub in the Manchester area, they were given to the 'bouncer' to sell. More used to having him deal with undesirable or disruptive customers, the entire clientèle found his attention focused on *them*. Far from ejecting them into the street, it seems he wouldn't let any of them leave the club unless they *bought a badge*! They were more or less imprisoned and the 'open sesame' was the bright yellow button. Maybe some bought them with the thought that it was worth 50p to get home (anything for a quiet life!). Others, having wined and dined at a cost of several pounds, maybe considered that another 50p was neither here nor there. Perhaps there were some who gave 50p – no matter what it was for! – rather than argue with a six feet four hunk of brawn and muscle who was determined to sell his allocation of badges. Whatever the reason, each went home 'One in a Million'.

In Blackpool, Lewis's Limited had kindly allotted counter

space near to the escalator on the ground floor to members of the Blackpool South Branch. For several days, Margaret Parkinson and her committee manned the counter and most people bought the badges willingly. There were however, a few exceptions.

One, I am told, was a lady wearing a mink coat, whose supercilious demeanour upset one of Margaret's helpers.

'What are you selling?' asked the lady, looking down an aquiline nose at the array of yellow badges.

Margaret duly explained.

'Oh, I'm not wearing one of those tin things,' replied the lady, somewhat disdainfully.

Margaret began to say that it wasn't that the badge itself was worth 50p. It was a way of giving a donation to the Fund . . . but before she could get the words out, her friends erupted with:

'Yes, and if you ever have reason to be in the Christie and in need of the scanner, that bloody fur coat'll do you a lot of good in your wardrobe, won't it?'

Looking rather shaken, the lady bought a badge and shoved it in her pocket.

'And I hope it burns a bloody hole in it!' muttered Margaret's irate friend.

A more willing customer who came into Lewis's was a man with only one leg. Some years previously, the other had been amputated to save his life, as it was cancerous. The operation had been performed at the Christie and the gentleman extolled the hospital's praises to anyone on Lewis's ground floor who cared to listen.

Some people hesitated to wear a badge that claimed they were one in a million. Some thought it seemed boastful. But for many who have worn our badges, they have often provided a talking point with complete strangers. Remarks have varied from, 'That's a big headed thing to wear, isn't it?', to, 'What makes you think *you* are one in a million?' Badges have changed hands – or lapels – for 50p, in railway carriages, on buses, in clubs, pubs and shops. Many supporters started carrying half a dozen in their purses or pockets, ready to sell to the people whose curiosity got the better of them. They were the source of many an exchange of wit and humour and sometimes, a source of embarrassment.

On the magistrates' bench one morning, my husband, along with two other JPs, was confronted with a defendant wearing one of the Fund's badges. As I remember, it was some minor traffic offence. Geoff conferred with the Clerk: 'Look, this chap is wearing one of the badges in support of my wife's Fund. D'you think I ought to stand down?' (If a magistrate knows a defendant, he has to declare the fact and withdraw from the bench.) The Clerk looked at the defendant, then said, 'Do you know him?'

'No, I don't.'

'Well get back up there. Half the town are wearing them. You can't stand down for everyone who comes into court wearing one of those!'

On 14th March, I spent the day in the Manchester area, visiting several factories. It was many weeks later when I heard this story. There were alterations and extensions being carried out at one of the factories I visited that day and a building firm had a foreman and a dozen men on the site. Because the manager of the factory knew I was coming, he wouldn't have anyone on the place who wasn't wearing a badge. That included not only his own staff, but those of the builder. I'm not sure whether it was the builder himself, or the foreman who turned up at the house of Jean Wootton. 'For God's sake, Jean, give me some of those bloody badges!' He pulled out his wallet and handed over the required amount. 'It's now half past ten and I've had all those men cooped up in their bloody hut since eight o'clock! They haven't done a stroke of work yet and Mr S— won't let them out unless they've got a badge! They're costing me money even before I've bought them.' He drove back to the factory, doled out the badges and the workmen emerged from their hut with them pinned to their donkey jackets – and work could begin.

Later, I heard that some folk were wearing *two* badges – to show they've given a pound to the Fund. And on an oil rig off the coast of Greenland, they really were sold at a pound apiece.

One of the most amusing stories about the badges came to my notice in July, when a lady wrote to me to say that our 'One in a Million' badges had saved her family from an aggravating hour at the end of a long journey.

'In the past, whenever we have gone on holiday abroad, we have never yet managed to get through British Customs without having to unload everything out of the car for inspection! This year, the Customs officer approached the car with that usual menacing look and asked me if I had anything to declare. I put on my most innocent face and answered that we had been most careful and that we had nothing over the limit. I was, however, getting ready to start unpacking. The Customs officer gave me another searching look and then glanced at my handbag which was displaying one of your badges. He said that if I was "One in a Million", I couldn't possibly be telling a lie – and with that, waved us on our way.

'Could this be a new selling point for your badges – to would-be smugglers?'

On that 14th March, the total was £497,809. The following day, the Fund would be just one year old. Would we crack the half million for the first anniversary? The following morning, the postman delivered a fair amount of mail, and as usual, the donations were entered and paid into Nat-West with all speed. Christine, Mr Ball's secretary promised to ring me as soon as that morning's bank clearing figure was available. About eleven o'clock the phone rang.

'You've done it. Here's your total – £509,776.'

Nearly £12,000 overnight. It was unbelievable. Where had it all come from? It had taken six or seven *weeks* to raise the first £12,000.

Time after time, throughout the Appeal, I have thought: 'After that, nothing will surprise me,' and then something else has happened and I've thought exactly the same again. This has happened so many times that it almost seems that the incredible has become the norm. I remember someone asking me, 'Don't you find yourself becoming blasé about all this money?'

Blasé? No. Never that. It has been interesting and gratifying to watch the total rise and to watch the progression rate fluctuate according to publicity or other factors. Admittedly, in some respects, the money is just an escalating set of figures. But it is a means to an all-important objective and I have never lost sight of the fact that each day's increased total is due to someone's efforts or some person's generosity. People have not only given money; they have given of themselves. There is no way that I could become blasé about that.

If the 15th March was a milestone for the Fund, the 17th was a milestone for me, in that I reached my half century. I told friends they could congratulate on the former and commiserate on the latter! Why does fifty sound so much older than forty-nine? However, I have never been coy about my age and far from being depressed, there was an understandable thankfulness.

There was no doubt that the Appeal and all it entailed was also good therapy for me. There was so much to do, so much of interest, some things to cry about and much to make me laugh. And above all there was friendship. But the pace was ever increasing and I was in need of help. Regular help. If fifty sounded old, I had to admit that there were days when I felt more like ninety and too tired to even think straight.

In March, I had only six evenings by my own fireside and some of those were spent typing. I was working a fourteen-, fifteen- or sixteen-hour day – enough to floor a fit person. It is only looking back that I realise just how great the pressures were and wonder if I could ever do it again . . .

For two to three months in late 1977, a good friend who is a first-class secretary had given me several hours of her time each week. Eileen would take my replies to letters down in shorthand and bring them back later, neatly typed, ready for signature. She was a Godsend. Then her husband became seriously ill, and understandably, she had to give up. Since then, I'd managed by myself, making sure the money was paid into the bank immediately, but answering letters as and when I could, when ever I was at home for a few hours each day. The Fund's treasurer put his foot down. He said that I was trying to do more than was humanly possible; the Appeal was well established and it was high time I had the help of a paid secretary. I was reluctant at first. I'd organised the whole thing on a voluntary basis and I wanted to keep it that way. Under no circumstances would I touch the capital. Mr Ball said that a small salary could be paid out of the interest and, the rate I was going on, I would be in no fit state to volunteer for anything.

'Pat, you're being ridiculous. You're running yourself into the ground. You are not being fair to yourself.'

'You sound just like my husband. He's been telling me that for ages.'

'You are not being fair to him, either. How much does he see of you, these days?'

'Not much, I admit, but he knows what I'm trying to do and he does everything he can to help me. This is a partnership, you know, not just a solo effort.'

'Even so, if the pair of you are going to stay the course, you must be more realistic. You've got to have some help.'

'I know, I know . . . but a lot of the letters I receive are confidential. They're not business letters. Some people put their hearts on paper. They tell me of their own difficulties and worries and most of them are cancer patients. Some are at their wits' end and write to me in desperation, hoping I'll understand or be able to help them . . . you couldn't show those letters to just anybody. If I have to have a secretary, I don't only need someone who is completely trustworthy: I also need someone with a sympathetic personality; someone who will respect confidentiality. These things are far more important to me than shorthand and typing speeds.'

Mr Ball agreed and a few days later rang to tell of his brain-wave.

Mrs Pauline Heaton, the wife of the headmaster of our local CE Junior School had been doing the clerical work in connection with the renovation of our parish hall under the government's Job Creation Scheme. The work was in its final stages. In another week or so Pauline would be free to take on other work.

Pauline has made life a lot easier for me, but there are still times when it takes the two of us all our time to cope. Times when the pressure is on and I still need to send out an SOS to friends, who come armed with their typewriters and give me as many hours as they can spare.

Pauline says, 'That phone of yours rings and you never know who it's going to be, or what is going to happen as a result.'

It rang one day in early April. The caller was Lynne Silver, a researcher for the Russell Harty Show produced by London Weekend Television. Could she come to see me to discuss the possibility of me appearing on the programme? We arranged that I'd meet her at Preston railway station a few days later.

I put the receiver back on the rest, came into the lounge and said to Pauline: 'Who's Russell Harty?'

'*Who's Russell Harty? Don't you know?*'

'How much time do I have to watch TV? I'm never in the place. Go on – tell me, who is he?'

She was incredulous

'You must be about the only person in Britain who doesn't know who he is!' She told me.

If I thought for a minute that conversation would upset Russell, I would not include it in this book. My guess is that it will appeal to his sense of humour.

When I met Lynne in Preston, we went to a local pub which puts on rather nice lunches. As we ate, we discussed the Appeal in detail. A couple of hours later, she caught a train back to London. Two days later, she telephoned to discuss dates. The programmes were recorded on Wednesday nights for screening on Friday evenings. On Wednesday 12th, I had promised to go to Rossendale, so we settled for 19th April.

'What shall I wear?'

'Oh, wear whatever you feel happiest in. The show goes out late at night so an evening dress would be fine if you have one.'

I did a mental flip through my wardrobe and discarded the lot. There were half a dozen evening dresses, most of which I'd made myself in the days before the Appeal, when I'd plenty of time for sewing. In normal circumstances, I make about seventy-five per cent of my dresses but the 'Scanner Trail' left little time for such homely occupations. I'd worn all of the evening dresses in my wardrobe many times at various functions during the past year. I was sick of the sight of them. It was time I had a new one.

Remembering a pattern I'd bought some time ago and not got around to using, I fished it out of my sewing drawer. Yes, it would do. On Garstang market, I bought some deep red material. But *when* was I going to make it?

'Why on earth don't you go and buy one,' said Geoff. 'Why do you have to do everything the hard way?'

'One – I begrudge paying astronomical prices for dresses I will only wear half a dozen times, and two – I hate trying clothes on in shops. It's harder work than working!'

The sewing machine almost seized up at the unexpected demands made on it. All day, it and I worked at full speed. By evening the dress, for better or for worse, was finished. All it needed was a final pressing and that was fitted in during a brief spell at home between Manchester and Lancaster the following day. For me, that dress seems to typify the Appeal. Oh it's nothing to write home about. Dior or Yves St Laurent are not likely to find themselves redundant. Maybe it's the colour, that of the red Lancastrian rose. Maybe it's the speed and the sense of urgency with which it was made which is synonymous with everything about the 'Scanner Trail'. I know that if I were to live to be a hundred and were to look back over the years to the events of this period, it's that red dress I would see. I know it's illogical and maybe just plain sentimental, but that dress reminds me of the warmth, the good heartedness and the kindnesses that resulted after I wore it for the first time on television.

It was beyond my strength to travel to London, take part in a TV Show and travel back again the same night. Roy Fisher, our dear friend, lent me his London flat. Geoff and I had stayed there many times, and this time, Pauline and I and Mr Ball's wife, Kay, came along. I was thankful that I would be able to rest and have a meal before going to the studios at South Bank.

As the three of us arrived in the foyer at London Weekend TV, large stills of various TV personalities lined the wall and Pauline said: 'That's Russell.' So this was the ogre . . . I thought he looked rather nice. The picture showed a rather handsome, frank, open face, suggestive of a strong personality. But he didn't look as though he was going to eat me for breakfast! When friends knew I was to appear on his show, they'd almost frightened the life out of me with remarks such as: 'You'll have to watch it. He can be very tough!', or, 'He can be very abrasive. You'll be given the third degree treatment!' Yet they all said they enjoyed his programme. Then they told me he was a Lancashire man, born in Blackburn and I stopped worrying. I said that in that case I'd nothing to be nervous about. And if he was as tough as they made out, he'd find he was talking with a Lancashire lass who could match him round for round if necessary. In any case, as there was nothing controversial in the subject matter, I couldn't see that there would be need or reason to get tough.

As things turned out, the original was far nicer than his picture and kindness itself. Oh yes, there was a quality I recognised. It was one I'd grown up with – northern directness, which can so often be mistaken for rudeness; the knack of asking the straight question and expecting a straight answer in return and impatience and persistence when one isn't forthcoming.

But before I met Russell, Lynne collected us from the foyer and I was taken to the make-up room. As my face was getting the treatment, a diminutive blonde in a white muslim dress came in, asking if it was all right to wear white. I asked who she was and the make-up girl told me she was Clare Francis. *Clare Francis?* The intrepid yachtswoman? My stars, she didn't look as though she should hold anything heavier than a fan, let alone haul a yacht over mountainous oceans in Force Ten gales! She looked as sweet and demure as any Victorian Miss and as dainty as the fairy on our Christmas tree. And yet, one *knew* there had to be a toughness, a resilience and great courage behind that deceptively petite feminine frame. Clare was also to take part in the programme. The third interviewee was Bronwen Nash, an orchestral bass fiddle player who was endeavouring to prove the instrument's potential for solo performance. Later, she demonstrated its capabilities expertly and melodiously, to piano accompaniment. And so the 'programme content' was three women, all doing their own thing and succeeding in spite of the odds against them.

Russell was to interview me first. During our brief conversation before we went on set, I said to him, 'Look, what do I do about this?' pointing to my 'One in a Million' badge. 'Would you prefer that I didn't wear it?' We conferred with the producer, who asked what it was. When I had explained, he thought for a minute, then said, 'You wear it; Russell can ask you what it is. You tell him – and then sell it to him.'

The programme was filmed before a sizeable studio audience. As well as Pauline and Kay, I had two other friends there to give me moral support, Esther Harrod of the *Daily Express*'s London office and her husband, Barry. For almost twenty minutes, Russell asked me question after question, expertly drawing me out and covering all aspects of the Appeal and my personal situation. As a journalist, I quickly appreciated that he is a first-class interviewer. He wasn't in the least aggressive and I enjoyed talking with him. Finally, he produced a 50p piece out of his pocket and I sold him my badge. My part of the programme being over, I could now relax and watch Clare and Bronwen take the 'hot seat'. But before Clare came on the set, there was a short break, during which the studio manager remarked, 'What a pity we can't all buy one of those.'

'Excuse me,' said a voice from the audience, 'we have some badges.'

My efficient secretary isn't a Guider for nothing. She'd come prepared with a bagful of badges, and within the space of five minutes she and Kay had sold the lot. Later, when Bronwen was interviewed, Russell said to her, 'I see you're wearing one of those things, too.'

The programme was to be screened in two days' time on London Weekend, Anglia and Scottish commercial TV channels. Granada, our north-west commercial channel, would not be screening it until July. I remember remarking to Pauline that maybe there would not be a lot of response until the programme was shown in the north. I could not have been more wrong . . .

The following morning, Kay and Pauline went to look at the pictures in the Queen's Gallery and I went to Fleet Street. That was when Jean Rook fixed me with her gimlet eye and I found myself trying to do justice with mere words to a story I regard as nothing less than a miracle. Even this account has the typical Appeal quality about it. I began writing in leisurely fashion during my summer holidays. In late October, I found that the publishers wanted the final draft of the manuscript by the end of January. The pressure was on again!

On Friday of that week, Pauline and I dealt with the mail. On Saturday, she was going with her headmaster husband and a party of his school children on a week's holiday.

'I feel awful leaving you to it. What if there's a lot of post as a result of the programme?'

'Don't worry, I've managed before. I'll take it as it comes. You go and enjoy your holiday. There are friends I can call upon if necessary.'

Sunday was a free day. It was the last I was to have for some time and in a way, it was the calm before the storm. The following morning, there was an avalanche of letters – 647 of them – and the Post Office took pity on our cycling postman and sent them up in the van. In succeeding days I stopped counting them after the first 3,000 letters, being too busy trying to answer them all. In fact, for over a week, it took me two hours each morning just to slit open the envelopes.

SOS to several friends . . . the dining room became an extra office with four typewriters on the table. For a fortnight Geoff and I ate our meals on the coffee table in the lounge, shifting piles of paper in order to do so. The lounge had typewriters on occasional tables and there were even people sitting on the floor, entering donations in NatWest paying-in books. Batches of these were taken to the bank and the receipts clipped to the letters until I had time to deal with replies. Any friend who turned up at my front door expecting to be entertained to coffee and a chat, found herself on the end of a pen, pressganged into helping. When Pauline came back, she pitched in, too, and it was more than a month before the pace began to slacken. During all this time, my little Mother kept us all going with cups of tea, cups of coffee and the kettle was never cold. A farmer friend brought his wife, a fellow Soroptimist, one day. He came in to see what we were doing and stayed the rest of the day to help. At lunchtime, he went to the fish and chip shop in the town and bought us all our lunch. He said it was the only way we looked like getting any.

At London Weekend, Patricia Heald, Russell's personal assistant, said that they also were inundated with mail and that they'd never known anything like it. I apologised for the extra work load I had caused them.

On Friday, 28th April, the original target figure of three quarters of a million pounds was achieved. That night, Geoff and I were asked to attend an event at Preston Grasshoppers Rugby Union Football Club. Geoff had been a member for as long as I'd known him. In our courting days, I'd watched him play, but whenever I did, he always seemed to end up at the local Infirmary having stitches inserted in his face, so I soon gave that up and left him to play the game without my moral support from the touchline. When his playing days came to an end, he ran the Colts team – boys of under nineteen – for about fourteen years. On Easter Saturdays, when the seven-a-side matches were played at the 'Hoppers, I, along with other wives, made mountains of sandwiches in an effort to cater for young healthy appetites. I have never seen food disappear so quickly.

On 28th April, club members were putting on their own entertainment in support of the Appeal Fund and as we have a lot of friends there, we were on home ground. The programme they'd devised was hilarious, with plenty of jokes about a rival Rugby Club; hulking six footers in drag and plenty of good talented turns. When the Chairman, Richard Eastwood, invited me on to the stage at the interval, I took with me a bottle of champagne, and told them why I was in a celebratory mood. Obviously, one bottle of champers wouldn't go round a club room of some two or three hundred people, so I invited the chairman and one representative from each team to share it with Geoff and me.

It was yet another milestone along the way and what *should* have been the end of the journey. Now, I knew it wasn't enough. It was like coming to the crest of the hill, expecting it to be the summit, only to find that beyond it, was another steep path, still to be trodden and another peak still ahead. Little did I know that there were several peaks still ahead, with the pace ever increasing.

The power of 'the box' is frightening. Donations to the Fund as a result of that one programme came to about £100,000. But the letters didn't only contain money. Suddenly, I had an army of unseen friends, all of them helping me, all of them wishing me well. I find it difficult to describe how I felt. They contained such overwhelming kindness and concern; they were full of encouragement, not only for the Appeal, but for my personal welfare. Some made me laugh, others made me cry, but I treasure them all and I have kept every one of them. They are in boxes, on the outside of each box is written in thick felt pen 'Russell Harty, April, 1978'. Among the letters were many requests for badges and many kind folk in the south and the eastern districts of England offered to sell them. Even the Bunny Girls at London's Playboy Club sold them for us. Yes, Julé's badge scheme was a huge success and to celebrate, Paddy had a 'One in a

Million' badge fashioned in gold for her birthday.

I think her brilliant inspiration is best summed up in the words of an anonymous London resident, who sent 50p in an envelope. Inside was a single piece of paper without either name or address and the only words on it were: A BLOODY GOOD IDEA.

You can say that again, chum, you can say that again . . . for the sale of the badges has added almost £175,000 to the Fund.

Alas, Julé wasn't to wear her gold badge for long.

I visited her on 2nd September. She was sitting propped up in a chair, looking as pretty as a picture. Marie had come with me. Paddy made us all a champagne cocktail and I showed Julé the plans for the new CAT Department. But we all of us knew that it was the last time that Julé and I would meet. All her treatment had been suspended and it was only a matter of time . . .

Julé died on 5th October and she was buried in her home town of Market Harborough. A wreath was sent on behalf of the Appeal Fund from the Christie. I asked that my personal floral token should be a circlet of yellow flowers and that the attached card should have those immortal lines of John Bunyan's hymn: 'Who would true valour see, let him come hither', as my tribute to a brave friend.

Julé had maintained a courageous cheerfulness and had thought of others, knowing full well that her personal battle against cancer was lost.

I am glad she knew how successful her brilliant idea had been and how magnificent the contribution. I am proud to have known her and called her friend. Like her badge, Julé Hayward was pure gold.

9

The High Places

My heart seemed to miss a beat as I looked at the envelope. I was apprehensive. I had an idea what it might contain. Geoff had brought it upstairs, along with a cup of tea and the rest of that morning's mail. On the front of the envelope in large bold type, were the words: 'From the Prime Minister'.

'Well, aren't you going to open it?'

'No, you open it for me.'

Geoff sat down on the edge of the bed and as I watched him slit the envelope and take out the letter, I sat there as one hypnotised.

'What does it say?' The suspense was awful.

He put his arms round me and kissed me.

'Bless you, love, it's no more than you deserve. You've earned it well and truly. Here – read it for yourself.'

The letter said that the Prime Minister had it in mind to recommend to Her Majesty the Queen that I be made a Member of the Most Excellent Order of the British Empire. He wished to be assured that such a recommendation would be agreeable to me.

Over the months I had received very many letters from people from many parts of the north-west, telling me that they had written to either the Queen, the Prime Minister or to their MP suggesting that I should be included in the Honours List. Much as I appreciated the sentiments they expressed, the thought of Her Majesty being bombarded with letters of this kind filled me with embarrassment.

'Well, how are you going to answer it?'

'Oh heavens, I don't know. I'd rather he'd had it in mind to give me £100,000 for this Fund. Geoff, you know I'm not looking for medals or pats on the back. I just want to get on with the job and see that scanner installed. That's the important thing.'

'I know love, but consider for a moment . . . if you turn it down, you'll be letting down an awful lot of people. You've always maintained that this isn't a one-woman Appeal. Don't you see? This is recognition for all the people who have backed you to the hilt, all the men, women and little children who've seen fit to follow your lead. The success of the Appeal is their achievement as well as yours. You are no more alone in this than in any other aspect of the Appeal.'

Of course. Put like that, I would accept it, gladly and with pride. Later, showing the Award to people at fund-raising functions I attended, Geoff's opinion proved so right. The silver medal on its coral pink and light grey ribbon bow was passed around, admired, tried on. Children were thrilled to wear it for a few minutes, or have their picture taken, wearing it pinned to their school blazers. It was a source of pride and pleasure. Everybody felt they had a share in it. The medal belonged to them and what is more, so did I.

A most poignant display of the MBE took place at Oldham when I showed it to twenty-year-old Stephen Bilyenskyj. At the age of sixteen, Stephen had lost his sight as a result of a mugging fracas. Undaunted, he'd supported the Fund by doing a sponsored swim which had raised more than £700.

There are more ways of seeing than with the eyes. In Oldham's Civic Centre, I took him by the hand. 'Come and have a look at it, Stephen. It's yours as much as mine.' I took it from its box and placed it in Stephen's hands. As his fingers felt the indentations and the texture of the silver and the ribbon, I described it to him. Watching his young blond head bent over the medal, and his expression of concentration and of pride, it was as much as I could do to keep my voice steady and matter of fact and to keep the tears from my eyes.

But this was later. On this April day, the matter was confidential. The Birthday Honours List would not be announced until Saturday, 3rd June, the Queen's official birthday.

The first rumblings – and I use the word advisedly – that the Award was about to become public knowledge, was on Thursday, 1st June. An editor friend, who is not especially noted for his melodious singing voice, telephoned. Over the wire came his rendering of the one time hit of Cliff Richard's, 'Congratulations'. I giggled and told Tom he'd be much better off sticking to journalism and that he'd never make the top twenty.

The Press generally get the List a couple of days in advance, with an embargo on publication until one minute after midnight on the Official Birthday. This gives us time to go through it, picking out local people and to do our homework in the form of potted biographies about the recipients. I knew the drill. I'd written any number of them myself.

Friday, 2nd June and in the morning's post a congratulatory card from my pals Len and John of the *Gazette*. 'A little dickie bird told us . . . all our love.'

A call from the *Daily Express* . . . 'We want a new picture of you for tomorrow. We don't have to tell you why . . .' No, they didn't and I steeled myself for yet another blaze of publicity. But I was quite unprepared to see myself smiling on the front page the next morning, with the accompanying banner headline 'Courage, MBE.' Was this *really* me? Was this how people regarded me? Later in the day, an enormous bouquet of flowers arrived from the Editor and staff of the

Manchester office of the *Express*. The flowers filled several vases and the sitting room looked like a bower. I later wrote a letter of thanks to the Editor, which they printed, omitting to mention the flowers.

From eight in the morning, the phone started ringing. The calls were non-stop and it was eleven before I managed to get bathed and dressed. One call was from one of my willing helpers (who shall be nameless) who had helped with the mammoth task of sending out those 7,000 letters to Industry and who had helped me to cope with the inflow of mail following the Russell Harty programme.

'Congratulations, old girl. You know what MBE stands for, don't you?'

'No. What?'

'More Bloody Envelopes!' It was said with feeling.

Some days later a letter arrived from a lady who had supported the Fund regularly, suggesting that MBE stood for Many Blessings Eternally. It was typical of the pleasure the Award seemed to give to a great many people, many of whom took the trouble to send me cards of congratulations. Branch committees of the Fund wrote or phoned to say how delighted they were. It generated much happiness. It was mine, it was theirs, it was ours. It belonged to us all. I was the one to whom the medal would be pinned, but as the recipient I was the representative of many thousands of people, without whom the Appeal would have been nothing, nothing at all. As it was, it gave us all a shot in the arm and a renewed determination to see the job through to its successful conclusion.

That afternoon, I was down to cover for the three papers the visit of Group Captain Leonard Cheshire, VC, DSO, DFC, to the North Lancashire Cheshire Home in Garstang. It was his first visit to the Home for nine years and since those early days of its existence, much progress had been made. From a tentative beginning, it was now well established with extensions having been added to the mellow old house. The grounds of Oaklands are a delight and on this sunny afternoon the spacious lawn in front of the terrace was bordered with stalls, groaning under the weight of produce of all kinds. The stalls were manned by the Home's support groups and there was a huge crowd assembled to hear the Group Captain and to support this, the annual garden party.

In his speech before opening the event, Leonard Cheshire said that disabled people had a significant contribution to make to society in spite of their handicaps. Later, as Geoff and I talked with him, I was proud to tell him of the Fair the residents and staff had held in support of my Fund. This, when the Home needed every penny it could raise for its own needs. It confirmed what he had just said, that physical disability did not exclude integration and participation in community affairs.

I remarked to Group Captain Cheshire that I had found the Appeal to be a very humbling experience, as well as a rewarding one.

'I suppose you will know what I mean?'

'Oh yes indeed. I know exactly what you mean,' he said. 'I should think your Fund keeps you very busy, doesn't it?'

'Yes, it does, although I do try to pace myself.'

'Oh, but you must. If you don't, you're tempting Providence.'

He turned to my husband.

'Does she pace herself?'

(*Oh dear! . . .*)

'No,' said my better half, 'Pat does everything flat out!'

I could have thumped him.

Leonard Cheshire then said that everyone needed periods of renewal. I should set aside certain hours of the day which were just for myself and I should guard them jealously. The advice echoed many similar homilies from Geoff who had repeatedly told me that it was impossible to give one hundred per cent of myself for sixteen hours of every day to the Fund.

. . . 'The trouble with you is that you never know when you've had enough. You never know when to call a halt. Half the time you're too busy to think how you feel and the other half you're too damnably tired to care. What use are you going to be to anyone if you end up in the Christie again? For heaven's sake, slow down. Tomorrow's another day . . .'

And now, here was a dedicated man of much wider experience than mine, giving much the same advice.

Geoff's advice was out of concern for me. I know I worry him. The trouble is, I'm a poor one at saying 'No' to people who are working so hard and with such enthusiasm in support of a cause I started. If they want me at their event and I'm not already committed, I feel I have a responsibility to be there. I do not take their support for granted. In that month of June, I had only four free evenings at home. The other twenty-six were spent haring around the north-west. Finally, it was my consultant who put the brakes on. He limited me to no more than three days a week on the 'Scanner Trail'. He said that physically, I was not giving myself a chance.

'If you want to be there to see that scanner in operation, you've got to take things easier.'

When my friends of the branch committees heard this, back came the comments, 'We quite agree,' or, 'About time you learned some sense!' or, 'What's the point of delegating responsibility to us and trying to do it all yourself?'

On the evening of 3rd June, Geoff and I attended a social evening in aid of the Fund at Poulton le Fylde. Coming home in the car some time around midnight, I reflected on the day's events.

Pat Seed . . . MBE . . .

'Life's a funny thing, isn't it?'

'Why?'

'Oh, I don't know. Here I am with letters after my name. I never thought I'd ever have any. I was hopeless at exams . . .'

'You've passed the hardest exam of all, love – life itself. It's the toughest school of the lot and you've come out of it with flying colours.'

I felt tears welling into my eyes, but before they could overflow, with that sense of humour I know and love so well, Geoff brought me down to earth with:

'Of course, you know that MBEs are responsible for the National Debt, don't you?'

I laughed. 'In that case, heaven help the Nation!'

We were still laughing as he turned the car into our drive. Our friend the butcher had delivered our Sunday joint and the dog's rations. Both were on the kitchen work-top and on the latter was pinned a note: 'Bonnie Seed, MBE – Marrow Bone Expert'.

It had been quite a day.

Ten days later on 13th June I had several appointments in the Manchester area. Mrs Lynn Lever, chairman of the Altrincham, Hale and Bowdon Branch, accompanied me.

Our first call was to the Borough of Trafford town hall at Stretford, where we met a most charming lady, Mrs Shirley Fink. In May, Shirley had completed her year of office as Mayoress of the Borough. The Appeal Fund had been her charity for the year and in the presence of some of the Borough councillors, she presented me with a cheque for more than £18,000 – an unprecedented amount, for mayoral charities usually average about £3,000–£4,000.

After coffee, pastries and biscuits and a pleasantly informal chat, Lynn and I came out of the town hall just as the clock was striking twelve noon. Our next appointment was at Levenshulme on the other side of Manchester, at half past one.

'Look, Lynn, I've got to find something to wear for the Investiture and heaven knows when I'm going to find a free day to do it. Do you think we've time to pop into town and see what I can find in Kendals?'

'There isn't much time. It's either that, or lunch.'

'Are you hungry?'

'Not particularly. I don't eat big lunches.'

'Neither do I. Right – blow lunch. Kendals it is.'

By the time we had driven into town and found somewhere to park the car, it was twenty to one as we walked into the dress department of Kendal Milne Ltd on Deansgate.

At one o'clock, I left the store with two dresses and a hat.

One was an everyday cotton dress and the other was THE dress – pink crimplene, with an accordion pleated skirt, bell-shaped sleeves and a tie neckline. The hat I had chosen was white, green and pink turban style. In order not to look like a stick of spearmint, I thought black accessories would be better than white, but there was no more time to look for gloves. I had tried on four or five dresses when Lynn had produced THE dress from one of the rails.

'How about this?'

It was plain, unfussy and yet it had a bit of style about it.

'That's the one. If that fits me, I'll have it.'

It did.

As we came out of the store, Lynn said that she'd never known clothes to be bought so quickly. We laughed.

'That's the story of my life! You'd have thought I could have had at least a morning choosing something to wear for Buckingham Palace, wouldn't you?'

However, I was quite happy with what I'd got. I had some black shoes and a black handbag, but during the rest of June no opportunity presented itself to buy some black elbow-length gloves. In desperation I ended up with a black dye and dyed a pair of my white gloves. There are more ways of killing the cat than choking it with butter . . .

Lynn and I just managed to get across town to the Express Dairies at Levenshulme for one thirty, where the girls handed over the proceeds of their sponsored walk. They were a grand bunch of lasses and they gave us tea and biscuits which we accepted gratefully in lieu of the lunch we hadn't had. Later, we visited a blouse factory and a kitchen exhibition, thus completing the day's itinerary. At about five thirty, Lynn caught a train back to Altrincham and I threaded my way through the rush-hour traffic of Manchester in the direction of the M61 motorway.

By Monday, 19th June, the Fund was steadily climbing towards the million. The way the money was coming in, my estimate was that it would top it by about Thursday. What was I doing on Thursday? My diary told me I was due to go to an infants' school in Cleveleys, near Blackpool. I had a feeling that this could be the donation that would take it over the million pounds. With my special regard for little children, I hoped it would be, but I had other engagements before then. That night at Lancaster Town Hall, Lancaster University Rag Committee were to present a substantial cheque; on Tuesday, a large donation from Garstang Ladies Auxiliary and later in the evening, at Knott End Golf Club, the Over Wyre Rotary Club were to present their cheque; Wednesday, Chorley Lions presented a cheque at an event in the Royal Oak Hotel, Chorley, and money was pouring into Garstang Nat-West from all sources.

On Wednesday, 21st June, the total was £997,809. Newspapers had telephoned. When did I think it would be? Whose would be the donation?

'I can't say for certain. I'm pretty sure it's going to be tomorrow. As soon as I know, I'll give you a call.'

On Thursday morning, Pauline and I entered donations as quickly as we could and she took them to the bank. The staff, meanwhile, had totted up money paid in at other branches which arrived through 'clearing', the bank's computer system. At 10.30 a.m. the balance was £999,876. At two o'clock, I had to be at Northfold County Infants School, where the children were repeating a part of their concert, staged to celebrate 'World Children's Day' and the cheque was £308·85. This was it . . .

There is nothing more delightful than watching small children perform. In the school hall, parents and staff were the audience and little ones dressed in the national costumes of various countries sang appropriate songs and recited relevant lines. There were those with plenty of confidence, who obviously thoroughly enjoyed taking part; there were the shy children for whom it was an ordeal and who struggled stoically through the parts allotted to them. Facial expressions mirrored their thoughts, but the concert was colourful, tuneful and endearing. When it was over, I was given the cheque, being the proceeds of their sponsored 'hush-in', by a little boy with a face like a Botticelli angel.

Thanking the children, I said how much I appreciated all that they had done to help me, but I was going to ask them another favour.

Two weeks earlier, at lunch with Blackpool Marton Rotarians, I had been given a huge stick of Blackpool rock, measuring four feet in length and seven inches diameter and which had my name right through it. I knew just the people to help eat this . . .

'D'you think you could help me?' and the whole school chorused, 'Yes!' *Gazette* photographer, Peter Emmett, a Marton Rotarian, carried in the stick of rock – far too heavy for me to lift – and the children's eyes widened when they saw it. In the school playground, the entire school assembled and national dailies and local papers took pictures of us. There followed a glass of champagne and a recorded telephone conversation with BBC Radio Blackburn, in headmistress Mrs Elsie Izod's office. Then Mrs Izod, with four of her pupils, Sasha, Philip, Darien and Byron in her car, followed Pauline and me in my car, to Granada's TV studios in Manchester.

A million pounds . . . I just couldn't take it in . . . but it was *there*. It was a landmark, a milestone.

Zooming along the M55 and the M61 at a rate of knots, a feeling of elation overtook me. Yippee! It was great! Fantastic!

There just weren't enough superlatives. I could have waltzed the car along the motorway, except that common sense or maybe a natural instinct for survival took over. Instead, Pauline and I sang 'Granada' at the tops of our voices, la-la-ing when we couldn't remember the words. If anyone had heard us, they'd have had us certified. I wouldn't have cared. This was a Red Letter Day, a never-to-be-forgotten day. The noise of the traffic drowned our renderings and I kept my eyes on the road with occasional glances in the rear view mirror to make sure Mrs Izod and the children were still with us.

We marched into Granada Television with the huge stick of rock, brandishing a large carving knife and an outsize mallet – and nobody batted an eyelid! In the Granada Reports studio, I explained to the producer and to presenter Bob Greaves that we were celebrating the Million in good old Blackpool rock, which was appropriate, as the fund had started in Blackpool and it was a Blackpool school which had taken it over the million. Would Bob like to declare it 'open'?

Yes, he would. Sitting behind the low table on which we had placed the rock and with the four children, still in their national costumes, between us, Bob and I discussed the progress of the Appeal. Finally, he poised the carving knife over the centre of the rock, gave it an almighty thwack with the mallet and it split neatly in half. He handed one half to Sasha and Philip and the other half to Darien and Byron. It was a nice piece of television journalism.

Back in Granada's hospitality room, we met another person who was to appear on the programme. Our part had been filmed, but Bootsie Collins, who, it seems, is around the top of the American Punk Rock scene, was to appear 'live'. The children's eyes nearly popped out of their heads when they saw this larger than life, six feet four coloured American singer. He was dressed in a cowboy outfit, complete with Stetson and high-heeled red boots – the whole lot covered entirely in red and silver sequins. A member of his entourage asked what we were doing there and we duly explained. 'Bootsie', toting a child's toy pistol, gave me one of his LPs to raffle for the Fund. The time was then about five fifteen and the programme was to be screened at six o'clock. As we ate sandwiches and drank tea, we watched rehearsals on the monitor screen. At about five minutes to six we heard a voice say: 'Somebody had better go and tell Pat and the children that they are not going to be on the programme.'

We looked at each other. What had gone wrong?

Two members of staff came to tell us that the cameraman had fed the film of a football match into his TV camera instead of a blank reel. The result was a double exposure and useless. Nor could we repeat the performance. You can't bash a lump of Blackpool rock in half, twice.

Sadly, we made our way to the car park. For myself, I was philosophical. You can't win 'em all . . . but I was so disappointed for the children. They, however, didn't seem unduly worried. They were more concerned about getting that rock back to Cleveleys. Just as we were getting into the cars, voices shouted, 'Come back. Come back!' Result – Bob interviewed me briefly, at the end of the programme. He's a nice guy and he also was upset for the children. But in any job, things don't go smoothly all of the time. That day, the gremlins were at Granada, although those watching the box would not have known it.

It was a milestone along the 'Scanner Trail' and a memorable day. It was also my father's birthday. In spite of the hectic pace, I had not forgotten to send him a card and to buy him a present. But he was so thrilled about the Fund, he couldn't have been more excited had somebody given *him* a million pounds. Someone – I forget who – suggested I should take over Denis Healey's job as Chancellor of the Exchequer. Geoff said, 'Why can't you manage your housekeeping money like that?'

*

The Grand Theatre, Blackpool . . . a beautiful example of an ornate Victorian theatre, on the stage of which famous artistes performed during many decades. Now, it is owned by EMI and used as a bingo hall to cater for the customers' current interests. At a cost of many thousands of pounds, EMI restored the theatre to its original decor. Every night of the week, it is filled with people who enjoy playing this game. Now and then live shows – midnight matinées – are put on at the Grand and this is when the fine old theatre comes into its own.

Bob Parsons, the manager, has spent years in show business and on the night of Monday, 26th June, he'd arranged a 'Super Star Night'. Ken Dodd topped the bill, special guest star was Colin Crompton, the compère was Peter Robinson and ten other well-known acts completed the programme. EMI had offered the use of the theatre free of charge, the staff of the Grand worked until the small hours of the morning without pay and the 'Friends of the Grand' (those who hope to restore the place to its former glory as a venue for live theatre, by purchasing it from EMI, if enough money can be found), did a great deal of voluntary work backstage. The theatre was packed.

Bob is a staunch supporter of the Fund and that night, he gave Geoff and me right royal treatment, asking the audience to stand as he welcomed us both on stage before escorting us to the Royal Box, which the irreverent refer to as 'the egg cup'. Because of the evening's bingo session, the show did not begin until eleven o'clock and it didn't finish until after three in the morning. The show never flagged. It was great. Not only because of the variety of talent – which there certainly was – but also because of the wonderful atmosphere, the aura of goodwill about the whole evening which was almost a tangible thing.

The only thing that went wrong was me.

During the past months, I had sat through Ken's act many

times, finding it just as funny, even though, by now, I knew more or less what was coming. I say more or less because he doesn't use identical material for every show. There are always new insertions and omissions. But I reckoned I knew when he was coming towards the end of his act, which is usually his song 'Happiness'. A couple of minutes before I thought this was due, I made my way out of the 'egg cup' down to the side of the stage and watched him from the wings.

In my hands, I had a small present for him, which I hoped he would like. What can you possibly buy for a man like Ken Dodd? There was nothing I could buy for him that he couldn't buy for himself. So I had painted two of my floral miniatures for him. He had given so much of himself for the Fund, I wanted to give him something I'd done myself. The paintings were my attempt to say 'thank you'.

What I didn't know was that Ken and his organist, Stan, had planned an extra item as a surprise for me. Before 'Happiness' Ken sang the old song 'Thanks a Million', looking towards the Royal Box as he did so – and I wasn't there. Everyone must have thought I'd gone home, for it was past 3 a.m. I didn't know whether I should sprint back up the stairs or stay put. Either way, I'd missed my cue.

There was a cheque for Clatterbridge, but this time, it wasn't given to Ken. Instead, I asked Mr Ron Walker, who is the liaison officer of the Fund, to escort on stage Mrs Kay Kelly.

I was glad to meet Kay again.

This memorable night ended with a final quip from Ken: 'When you see the Unigate man on your way home, ask him where he's been until now!'

The dawn was breaking over the hills as we headed back towards Garstang.

'What's the betting it comes bang in the middle of our holidays?'

'If it does, it does. We'll cross that bridge when we come to it,' said Geoff.

We were speculating on when the Investiture might be. We had become philosophical about time off. Whenever we planned something, it never seemed to work out as we'd hoped it would. Either the exhaust fell off the car or the weather decided to give a repeat performance of Noah's Flood. This time, we'd planned to have a fortnight's family holiday at Trearddur Bay, Anglesey. We were to rent a friend's flat. Just four miles from Holyhead, Trearddur was the scene of five sun-soaked summer holidays shared with Roy and Kay when their children and ours were small. In those days we had rented houses which were big enough to sleep a regiment and we invited all and sundry to come to stay, with a largesse which often meant that Kay and I felt as though we were catering for the five thousand.

But it didn't matter. Trearddur never let us down. The sun always shone, the sea offered a sparkling invitation and the kids ran wild. For us, Trearddur was the nearest thing to paradise and the location of many happy memories. We were looking forward to seeing it again, to getting off the 'Scanner Trail' for a while and to being just a family, with no letters, phone calls or callers to distract us. We had arranged to spend the first two weeks of July there and I intended to use the remainder of my month off to catch up on household chores which had been niggling me for some time. Things like washing the curtains, etc. Then came the letter to say that the date of the Investiture was to be 12th July. We decided that rather than make a fuss by asking for an alternative date, we would curtail our holiday and accept the date we had been given.

I could take two guests. I decided that as well as Geoff, I would like my mother to be there. Mum had done so much to help keep the domestic scene going, leaving me free to charge about all over the north-west to attend functions in aid of the

Fund. At seventy-seven, Mum wasn't likely to have another opportunity to go to Buckingham Palace.

She has always been an ardent Royalist, ever since, like many women of her generation, she had first had a crush on the young Prince of Wales who later, as Edward VIII, had abdicated the throne to marry Mrs Simpson. For my generation, the Duke of Edinburgh is our Royal pin-up. Michael and Helen had the rest of their lives for such opportunities. They were young enough; Mother wasn't.

A few days before we were due to go away, Mother started with shingles. I wanted to cancel our holiday but she wouldn't hear of it. 'What could you do if you stayed? You need this holiday. Go on, get yourselves off. Shingles will take their course and there's nothing you can do.'

Pauline and Marie promised faithfully to call at her home each day to make sure that my parents were coping and I arranged to ring one of them each day to make sure. I would also ring Mother every day and if I was needed, I'd come home at once.

Geoff was to pick up Helen and her husband Gerard and their baby at their Liverpool flat and Mike and I and Bonnie travelled in my car. We had just got it packed up, with Mike and the dog, plus his basket, already in the car when the telephone rang.

'Go on, get on your way or you'll never make the break!' Pauline more or less shoved me through the front door and we fled.

In spite of cool northerly winds, Trearddur was heaven and every bit as lovely as we remembered it. For nine days we did nothing except enjoy each other's company. The rest of the family did plenty of walking, I gathered flora from rocks and shore and painted them. We lazed, read books, toured the island, revisiting old haunts, and at night, played Scrabble. Albeit only nine days instead of fifteen, it was the break we needed.

Meanwhile, Mother was progressing, but still far from fit. It was a toss up which would upset her most – taking her to London or telling her she wasn't well enough to go. Finally we left the decision to her doctor, who gave his permission and a supply of pain killers.

Journalist Alan Bennett travelled down with us on 11th July and that evening we invited him to visit us at Roy's London flat, for Geoff and Alan had discovered a mutual interest in Rugby Union Football.

As the train drew into Euston station and we unloaded ourselves and our cases on to the platform a fellow passenger smiled at me and asked: 'Are you Pat Seed?'

I said that I was.

'I saw you on the Russell Harty programme. I'd like to give you a donation.'

He took out his wallet and handed me some money and I thanked him.

Looking at the yellow badge in my lapel, he added, 'And I'd like one of those, too.'

'With pleasure – here, have mine.' I unpinned the badge and gave it to him.

Indicating the note in my hand he said: 'That *will* go in the Nat-West, won't it?'

'Most certainly. If you'll let me have your name and address, I'll send you the receipt.'

But the gentleman declined to identify himself. On the bank statement of the Fund for 14th July is an entry: Mr Smith – Euston – £5.

The Press cover Investitures on a rota system. Alan had asked for a pass to the inner quadrangle, but somehow or other, the following morning he was in the state ballroom to see the whole Investiture. Don't ask me how he managed it, but he did.

I have been asked many times if I enjoyed the Investiture and if I am truthful, the answer is 'no'. It is nobody's fault but mine. I was far too nervous. I am not always steady on my feet and I was terrified of falling flat on my face when I tried to curtsy; too apprehensive and praying that I wouldn't let the side down.

We drove through the Palace gates, under the arch into the inner quadrangle and under the porticoed entrance. That was where Geoff and Mother left me and I was on my own, for the arrows directed guests to the left and recipients to the right. The guests were ushered into the rectangular ballroom, with the throne at one end and the minstrel gallery at the other. Around three sides of the ballroom are tiers of red plush seats on which the guests are seated and on the ballroom floor are chairs on which those being invested sit, after receiving their award. The decor of the entrance hall, the grand staircase and of the ballroom is red, white and gold. It is immaculate.

Following the arrow 'recipients' I entered the hall and was approached by an usher.

'Which award, Madam?'

'MBE'.

He raised his hand and indicated the white marble staircase with its thick pile red carpet.

'At the top of the stairs, turn right and there'll be someone there to direct you.'

I ascended the staircase, passing at intervals Guards of the Household in flawless uniforms, standing sentinel with a practised immobility reminiscent of Tussauds. I turned to the right and another gentleman asked 'which award' and then directed me 'through those doors and keep to the right'.

'Those doors' were the huge mirrored doors leading into the long gallery, which was sectioned off with gold stanchions and thick red cord. An 'S'-shaped hook was attached to my dress and I was told in which section I should wait. There were already a large number of the 150 civilians and service personnel present, who were to be invested. It was with some relief that I saw a familiar face and made a beeline for Clare Francis. She, also, was to receive the MBE and was somewhat disturbed to find herself the only woman without hat and gloves.

'Would you like me to find my mother and borrow her gloves for you?' I offered.

'No, it's too late now,' said Clare, and then, looking at the partitioned long room, with OBEs in one section, MBEs in another and those to be invested with higher orders at the far end of the room, she said: 'It's like sheep pens, isn't it?'

We looked at the Rubens, Rembrandts and other pictures lining the walls.

'What do you suppose this lot would fetch at Sothebys?'

'I don't know – a lot of money!' said Clare.

We agreed that *that* was the last thing we would want to see happen to them and that too many of our art treasures had already gone to overseas buyers.

The masterpieces on the walls of Buckingham Palace are an irreplaceable part of our national heritage and, as such, it is a collection of which to be proud.

The Lord Chamberlain then called our attention. He gave us clear and detailed instructions about the procedure. With the higher orders taking precedence, we were taken to the ballroom in groups of ten or twelve. One could watch three or four people ahead of one making their bow or curtsy to Her Majesty and I saw Clare receive her MBE. The Queen wasn't wearing a hat or gloves, either. But then, why should she, in her own home? She was wearing a pink and lavender small patterned floral dress with an accordion pleated skirt and collar and on her feet were a sensible pair of low-heeled cream shoes – the latter essential, I should think, when one has to stand for about an hour and a half, investing 150 people.

And then it was my turn.

Please don't let me make a fool of myself. I must do this properly.

184

My name was called . . . Patricia, Mrs Seed . . . and my legs felt as though they didn't belong to me.

Five paces forward, turn left to face Her Majesty . . . curtsy . . . (*thank God I didn't fall*) and three paces to the foot of the dais.

Petite and charming, one is very mindful that this gracious lady is Queen of Great Britain and the Commonwealth. One is also conscious of the fact that she works as hard, if not harder, than any of her subjects. In her presence, one's affection and respect are renewed.

But what Her Majesty looks like at close quarters I honestly could not tell you. With her head no more than a few inches away from mine as she pinned on the MBE, my powers of observation deserted me as nervousness took over.

'I hear you've been raising money for charity,' said the Queen.

'Yes Ma'am, for the Christie Hospital, Manchester.'

'Oh?'

'People have worked awfully hard, Ma'am. I've been very fortunate to see so much of the good side of human nature.'

'That's very good to hear,' replied Her Majesty.

She then proffered her hand and gave me a smile of dismissal. Two paces backwards, curtsy again, turn right and leave the ballroom. In the passage beyond, the medal was removed from my dress and placed in its leather case and handed to me. The hook was put in a box along with others, ready for the next Investiture. Sitting on one of the seats on the ballroom floor, I could see nothing other than the heads of those in front of me.

The Guards' band in the gallery had been playing light music throughout the entire proceedings and one knows the whole thing is over when they strike up the opening chords of the National Anthem.

The Queen has gone, the Investiture is ended.

I made my way through the crowd to where Geoff and

Mother were sitting. Bursting with pride, they had gripped each others' hands as the Queen invested me and my mother vowed that Her Majesty had spoken with me for longer than with anyone else (of course she hadn't!). I said that they had seen more of the Investiture than I and commented that it was the onlookers who see most of the game. Then it transpired that Geoff had left his distance glasses back at the flat and my little Mum who is only four feet eight inches tall, had only seen the top of the Queen's head.

I came to the conclusion that none of us was fit to be let out.

Back at home, there was a letter from Tess with those gorgeous Solomon Islands stamps plastered on the envelope. Among her news of her adventures in those far-flung coral islands was the message, 'Congratulations, old bean. Have you washed those mucky curtains yet?'

10

Some Travelling Companions

So many things have happened during the last two years that my mind is crowded with memories. There are so very many stories behind the Appeal. Heartwarming, heartbreaking and hilarious, together they span the gamut of human emotions and endeavour.

It would be impossible to recount them all, but I include some, in the hope that collectively they will convey to the reader some of the many facets of the Appeal and of the spirit which emerged as a result.

Starting near to home, there's my friend Jack Benson . . . Jack is a man whose considerable artistic talents are handicapped by his easy going nature, his love of company and his liking for Boddington's bitter. They say one can insult one's friends. One is icily polite to one's enemies. If it's any indication of our friendship, I have to admit that I insult and bully Jack unmercifully – in repeated attempts to get him to settle down to *write*. Jack is by no means work-shy. He's a country window cleaner, but he's also a writer of verse, a singer of songs and a teller and a writer of tales. The latter, when you can pin him down. He's a solo performer and also a member of The

Cannyfowk, a local folk singing group who are very much in demand and who have raised many hundreds of pounds for various charities. I first met Jack, his charming wife Patty and their three little daughters several years ago when I was writing a feature about the Cannyfowk. This tall, gangling, bearded, bespectacled lad is one of the most likeable people one could meet. His ready wit, lack of pretentiousness and his nifty turn of dialect phrase ensure that he's never short of company. He's the sort of fellow who hasn't an enemy in the world.

As a writer of verse, he'd had several contributions accepted by *Lancashire Life* magazine. Then he decided he'd like to extend his talent to short story writing. His daily contact with the local community provided him with some excellent, original material.

Jack spent many an evening at our house and as he'd recount some unlikely anecdote in between swigs of Geoff's best export bitter, I'd say to him: 'Why don't you get that written down?'

'I'd get run out of the place if I put *that* in print!'

'Yes, I know you would in its present form. Change the circumstances, but use the situation. You've a good story line, there.'

'Aye, I will do, sometime,' he'd reply amiably, taking another draught of ale.

Hence the bullying. Eventually, he turned up with some Lancashire dialect stories for me to read, which I ruthlessly – and I hope constructively – criticised and made him rewrite. When they were accepted by *Lancashire Life*, I felt that at last I was getting somewhere with Jack Benson and I couldn't have been more pleased had the stories been my own.

From the start of the Appeal, Jack and the Cannyfowk had put on several concerts to raise funds and I appreciated all that they had done to help, but one anecdote of Jack's had me in stitches.

One morning, he telephoned me.

'Eh! I've got a tale for you.'

'Go on,' I said, 'let's hear it.'

'Well, I'm not telling you *who* it is, *when* it is or *where* it is, but a woman has just rung me up and she hasn't done a damn thing for my ego.'

'Why? What has she done?'

It seems Jack had been tucking into his toast and some of Patty's homemade marmalade when the phone rang. A bright voice had said: 'Oh, good morning, Mr Benson. We're holding a supper dance for the Pat Seed Fund. We would be so thrilled if you could come to do a cabaret spot for us.'

The lady mentioned the date and Jack checked his diary.

'Yes, all right.'

'Oh, Mr Benson, I'm delighted that you can make it. I can't wait to tell the others. They'll be so pleased.'

Jack said that at this point, he practised his modest smile.

The lady gushed on.

'We're all so looking forward to seeing you. What is it that you do?'

'Eh?'

'In your cabaret act?'

'Didn't whoever recommended me tell you what I do?'

'No. They hadn't seen you either.'

The modest smile sagged and fell apart.

'Then why have you asked me?' *There must be some reason, thought Jack.*

'Well, I did hear you'd come for nothing,' said the lady.

Jack's marmalade began to taste bitter and he said that he should have left it at that, but some devil in him persisted.

'But if you don't know what I do, how do you know that your audience will like me?'

'Don't worry about that, Mr Benson. I'll tell them you do it for nothing so they mustn't expect too much. Good morning.'

I was helpless. When I could speak, I said: 'And what are you going to do when you get there – sing that song of yours, "There's nowt so queer as folk"? On the other hand, you could always ring her back and tell her you've just had a booking from the London Palladium!'

'Aye, love, and I'd appear there for nowt, if it was for your Fund.'

As fans of the Cannyfowk, Geoff and I had attended a concert in which they'd taken part at Preston Guild Hall. Built to commemorate the 1972 Preston Guild, the hall is of modern design, seating about 2,000 people, and the acoustics are first class. Jack had commented that he could easily get stage struck, appearing on that stage.

'Why don't you put on your own folk concert then?' I suggested. 'You could make a bob or two for the Fund while you're about it. We'd all have a good night out.'

Jack said he couldn't organise a bun fight, let alone a full-scale concert, but he knew someone who could. The next day, he rang Eddie Green. Eddie builds top-quality guitars, is a teacher of the instrument and co-author of one of the best guitar manuals on the market. An accomplished musician who has the respect of the entire 'folk' world, he and his wife Anne are also first-class organisers. Before you could say 'knife', they'd arranged a Folk Night at the Guild Hall, with Bernard Wrigley topping the bill and with Strawhead, Dave Walters, the Cannyfowk and Jack Benson all helping to ensure that the audience got their money's worth. Brian Dewhurst, who had already donated the proceeds of one of his single records to the Fund, was to be compère and a recording team from Radio Blackburn were coming along to put the programme on tape.

Meanwhile, Jack was having a bit of a fight with himself. He says that when writers begin to talk about their work having deep inner meanings, or being deeply significant, he heads for the nearest bar. As a writer and teller of tales, usually humorous and often rude, he writes what he likes, when he likes. But for some time, he'd been feeling restless because he knew that there were things that he wanted to say about me and he'd get no peace with himself until he'd got them off his chest. He was to tell me later, 'No one had ever really portrayed the stark gut courage involved or grasped the personal enmity you feel towards cancer. It is almost as though you regard cancer and its lesser henchman, fear, as people; malignant beings to be fought and conquered.'

One Sunday morning, Jack locked himself away with a fistful of pens and a pile of scrap paper. By teatime, he was ankle deep in discarded scribble, but what my dear friend had written for me moved me to tears when I read it. Later, it was to be published in *Lancashire Life*, but in November 1977 he recited it at the Guild Hall concert. As he did so, the indicators on the BBC's audience noise monitors were on zero – a thing which rarely happens. There wasn't a sound in that huge auditorium as Jack Benson recited the following lines. And when he'd finished, there was hardly a dry pair of eyes in the place.

> The grey shadow turned and uncovered his head.
> With a terrible smile, 'I am Cancer,' he said.
> 'I'm the curse of Humanity down through the years,
> A taker of lives and a bringer of tears.
> You can't stand against me whatever you do,
> So weep now, Pat Seed, I come here for you.'
>
> Pat wept, as she must, at the weight of the blow.
> Then raising her eyes to that face, she cried 'No!
> I know you can maim and I know you can kill,
> But I know I can fight you and by heck, I will.
> I'll fight for myself, and if my chance be gone,
> I'll fight then for others who may follow on.'
>
> Cancer grinned, a grimace dreadful to see.
> 'You, little woman? You dare defy ME?'

'I dare,' replied Pat. 'For a long time I've known
That for all of your bragging, you don't fight alone.
You have an accomplice who always rides near;
A partner in darkness – and His name is Fear.

He rides on ahead and when his work is done
Your battles are over before they've begun.
Fear also can kill and fear also can maim;
Fear makes us reluctant to mention your name
And keeps sufferers silent at such dreadful cost.
If we destroy Fear, without him, you're lost.

We'll drag you out in the clean healthy light.
We'll see you – and what we can see, we can fight.
Then, with all the resources that science can lend
We'll not only fight you, we'll beat you my friend.'
Cancer spoke then: 'Your plan's expensive and rash.
For ambitions like these, you're going to need cash.

Your Government won't give you so much as one note.
The victims of cancer don't have a block vote.'
'I'll have help,' said Pat, 'for I won't rest until
I start such a move among folk of good will
That will grow to a landslide of kindness one day
And gather momentum and sweep you away.'

And so it may prove, for that one tiny start,
That fierce blaze of courage in one woman's heart
Has nurtured a rosebud and blossomed a rose.
On the goodness of good folk it prospers and grows.
And from we who have tried, Pat, to follow your lead,
Here's thanks, luck and love to our Pat – Our Pat Seed.

I was in the Christie administration office one morning,
following my monthly medical check, when one of the staff
came in. He had just returned from visiting an elderly lady in
the Stockport area, whom he described as an incredible
woman. As he told us the story behind his visit, I could only

agree with him and I determined that at the first opportunity, I would go to see her. This was how I came to meet Mrs Minnie Hall.

On 18th January 1978, I attended a Festival Concert at the Salvation Army Citadel, Stockport, an enjoyable event which raised £225. Here, I met Mrs Mollie Malpass, who had arranged the event and also Mr and Mrs Wallace Barber, I found that Mrs Hall was also a Salvationist, and a friend of theirs, but at the age of eighty-seven, she was now house-bound and had been for the last two years. We arranged that I would call on her at the first opportunity, which was on 22nd March.

Minnie lives alone in a ground-floor council flat in Edgeley on the outskirts of Stockport. She manages to get by with help of her good friends and neighbours, who see to her daily wants and needs. Minnie had brought up three children who were all now married, with children of their own, and she had been a widow for some time. Thirty years ago, she had a colostomy, but it hadn't prevented her from leading an active, useful life with the Salvation Army, until Father Time began to put the brakes on. Now, she was confined to a wheelchair. Even so, Minnie wanted to do something to help the Fund. Anyone could be forgiven for wondering what on earth a woman in Minnie's position could possibly do to help. But then, you would not have taken into account this indomitable old lady's unquestioning Faith and her conviction that human beings have a divine right and duty to help each other. Where there's a will there's a way. Minnie put a notice of the Appeal in her living-room window to attract the attention of passers-by. And as people walked past on the way to the shops, she'd rap on the window, open it and suggest that they put some money in her 'Pat Seed' tin. She enlisted the help of local school children, for she is the kind of old lady who has an easy rapport with the young. The children not only ran errands for her, they also brought donations – either from little efforts they'd held themselves, or from adults who used them as miniature messengers. When the officer from the Christie had called to see her, she had handed over a cheque for £200. Since then, her total has mounted to almost £600 and it's still rising.

I enjoyed my cup of tea and chat with Minnie. She inspired and encouraged me and I am proud to call her my friend. It is people like Minnie who make one realise that no human being need ever feel that they are of no use to anyone. Minnie's living room, with her presiding in her wheelchair, is the heart and hub of the neighbourhood. Whenever I am in the Stockport area and time will allow, there is nothing I like better than to spend a half hour in her company. I come away feeling renewed and refreshed by the unstinting generosity of this Christian soldier's spirit.

'How would you like to come to a frog race with me tonight?'

'*A what?*'

'A frog race.'

'What on earth's a frog race?' asked Marie, incredulously.

'Don't know. We'll find out when we get there.'

The evening had been arranged by the Blackburn Greys Ladies Circle, of which Mrs Lilian Hargreaves, who is chairman of the Blackburn Branch of the Appeal Fund, is a member. The night's proceeds were for the Fund.

Lilian had, of course, given me explicit directions.

'When you get to the roundabout, take the exit signposted "Burnley". At the first set of traffic lights, turn right and the hall is just down the road on the left.' She added, 'You can't miss it.' Famous last words . . .

Marie and I set off in the pitch dark night and all went well until we came to the roundabout in question. The first exit was signposted 'Burnley' and we headed along this road until we came to traffic lights, at which we turned right. The road then became a steep uphill gradient. It went on, and on, and on. We passed what we later discovered were the Wilpshire reservoirs and *still* the road twisted and climbed.

'This can't be right, surely?' I queried anxiously. 'There isn't a sign of a hall!'

The journey began to assume Everest proportions. Eventually, at the crest of the hill we came to a pub, the New Inn. As we got out of the car, the view was similar to that from an aircraft, for we could see round 360 degrees.

Nestling in the valleys, the sodium lights of several east-Lancashire towns illuminated these centres of habitation. In the pub, customers helpfully gave us directions, laughing good humouredly at our dilemma and telling us where we'd gone wrong. It seems we should have taken the *second* exit at the roundabout, which was also marked 'Burnley', the first road being only a 'B' road. Lilian couldn't have known she was directing someone who is an utter fool at navigation and an expert at getting lost.

Back in the car, we continued on our way, the gradient descending steeply until we came to the traffic lights at which we *should* have turned right. From then on, it was simple – except that we arrived half an hour late.

Inside the hall, Marie and I were given a warm welcome and a drink. The frog race was in full swing. With thoughts of cock fighting in my mind and visions of real live frogs being prodded into jumping in all directions, it was a relief to find that they were made of cardboard.

The idea is this: There are six cardboard frogs with long lengths of string threaded through them, lined up at one end of the room. Each 'frog' is auctioned and the highest bidders are the 'jockeys'. The jockeys have to jiggle the string to make the frog move towards them. There is a tote and the assembled company bets on the frog they think will reach 'home' first. The jockeys are egged on by the betters, who shout words of encouragement and who are not backward in coming forward with either constructive or useless advice. It's great fun. What is more, it raised a goodly sum for the Fund.

The Circlers made us very welcome and one of them made my night.

During the evening, a lady whom I will call Sheila came to talk to me.

'You don't know what you've done for me.'

'I don't think we've met before, have we? What have I done?' I asked.

'Well, I suddenly discovered a lump in my breast and I was terrified. I didn't want to tell anybody and I felt as though I was living in a nightmare. Then I thought of you. I thought to myself, "Damn it, if she can face up to cancer, so can I." I went to see my doctor, who sent me to a specialist and I've had a mastectomy. It seems it was a very tiny tumour and they're ninety-nine per cent certain that I'll have no further trouble. Of course, I'll have to go for check-ups periodically, but the point is this; but for you and the way you've brought cancer out into the open, I know that I would not have had the courage to go and get help. I just wanted you to know and I wanted to say "thank you", Pat.'

Oh, Sheila, you couldn't have pleased me more, had you given me a gold clock. After all the weeks and months of talking, persuading, encouraging those with any doubts to go and ask for help, this was reward indeed. In trying to remove fear, if it had meant that *just one person* had overcome it and done the sensible thing, it made all my efforts worth while. Why is it, that when something moves and pleases you so much, you find yourself close to tears?

Some time later, Marie and I headed instinctively and unerringly back to Garstang like a couple of homing pigeons.

I must tell you about my anonymous postman – he's a sweetie. But before I do, perhaps this is an appropriate place to say something about The Post Office. The staff of our local sorting office have come in for a considerable amount of extra work because of the Appeal. They must have delivered hundred-weights of mail to me and have coped with a similar quantity I have sent out. It has all been done with cheerfulness and helpfulness. And the postal service in general? Envelopes with the obscurest of addresses have arrived safely. Pat Seed, Garstang, Lancs . . . often, envelopes have been addressed to Garston, near Liverpool. That's one of the easier inaccuracies. 'Somewhere near Manchester' – more difficult perhaps? But for delivering a letter from abroad, marked 'Pat Seed Cancer Fund, England', they almost deserve a medal. I think there must be a few Sherlock Holmeses employed by The Post Office. Which ever way one looks at it, The Post Office have done a magnificent job for me.

But back to my anonymous postman. The only clue I had to his identity was the address, 'Rossendale, Lancs'. His first letter read: 'Hello Pat, Here's an afternoon's overtime towards your fund from a postman. Good luck. God be with you.' I sent the receipt to the Rossendale sorting office. Some months later, he wrote: 'It's that postman again – here's your share of our PO football pool. I won it at last, after about five years! Still think of you and praying for you and the Appeal.'

Howard Reynolds of the *Sunday Mirror* had called to see me with a view to writing an article. He's a thoroughly nice chap, who some years ago had worked for the *Lancashire Evening Post* in Preston. Over a cup of tea, we talked 'shop' and about the Fund. An hour or so later, he went away with a notepad full of information and quotes. When he'd written it up, he rang to check with me to ensure he'd got all his facts right. But the following issue of the *Sunday Mirror* contained an insignificant, single-column piece of no more than three inches. Short of space, some sub-editor had cut Howard's story down to the bare bones.

He telephoned to apologise and I giggled.

'Are you crying in your beer?'

We decided that most sub-editors ought to be impaled on their own spikes (that's what happens to copy which doesn't get into print) and Howard said he was thankful that he didn't have to explain to a member of the public what had happened to the article. At least, I understood the vagaries of the profession. I said that the only bit I objected to was that the piece had stated that I had raised the money 'single-handed'.

'That's a figment of someone's imagination. What are the fifty branches of the Appeal going to think, when they read that?

The following Sunday, 4th December 1977, the *Mirror* more than made up for it. They published a rewrite of Howard's article, quoting several examples of fund raising and donations, including those of my anonymous postman. It brought another letter from Rossendale. 'I see I made it in print. Here's another donation – more worth while this time – from friends and relatives. Still praying for you – The Postman.'

Early in 1978, Mrs Rita Goodwin, chairman of the Rossendale Branch of the Appeal, rang to tell me that there was to be a concert in aid of the Appeal in Rossendale on Wednesday, 12th April.

Could I come?

I said yes, I'd be delighted to come.

'Rita, do you think you could do something for me?'

'Certainly, if I can.'

I told her about my anonymous postman. 'He intrigues me. He sounds so nice. The last donation was by cheque, not postal orders. The signature was X— D'you think you could find him for me? I'd love to meet him, if he doesn't mind. On the other hand, if he prefers to remain anonymous, I'll respect that.' A week or so later, Rita rang to say: 'I've found your postman. He'll be at the concert.'

And that was how Geoff and I met Mr X— and his wife, a most kindly couple and he was just as I had imagined him to be, just as nice as he had seemed in his letters.

The concert was first class with some very talented singers and artistes putting on a most enjoyable programme. It was good to meet Rita and her husband again and to meet the other members of the Rossendale committee and their helpers.

But my anonymous postman made my night. There have been many anonymous donations. I know that this is how a lot of people prefer to donate to charity, but they do deny one the opportunity to say thank you.

In this respect, Mr X— was the one who didn't get away!

One day during the summer of 1978, the chairman of another of the branches telephoned, to tell me of a young man whom I will call Frank. It seemed Frank was a cancer patient and he was a terminal case. He had asbestosis – cancer of the pleura (which is the outer bag of the lung), caused by the fibres of asbestos. His doctors had estimated that he had about three months to live.

Married, with two young children, Frank was now back at home. This tragic situation was made even harder for his family because Frank was spending his time in his bed, curled up in a foetal position, refusing to see members of his family or his friends, with the exception of his wife.

'D'you think I could be of any use? Would it help at all, if I went to see him?'

'I don't know,' said my friend. 'You might come away with a flea in your ear. Maybe it's worth a try. I'll ask his wife and see what she thinks.'

Frank's wife was consulted and she said yes, she thought he might be willing to talk to me, but I must be prepared for a rebuff.

One sunny Saturday afternoon, my friend and I arrived at their cottage. Two young children were playing in the garden. Frank's wife greeted us and showed us into the kitchen, where we talked for some time about the family circumstances.

She said Frank had withdrawn into himself. The only person he'd have in the bedroom was her. His friends had been to see him and got nowhere with him. In fact, he'd told her they hadn't to come again.

'He's just lying there and he's so bitterly resentful. I wish there was something we could do.'

'It's a fearful shock to be told that you're dying, love,' I said, gently. 'It takes an awful lot of adjustment. *You* are under a tremendous strain as well, you know.'

'I know. I can cope with that. The thing is, he's so little time left and I want his last weeks to be as happy as possible. At the moment, he's not in too much pain.'

'Well, dear, I don't know whether anything I can say will make any difference, I can but try.'

My friend waited in the kitchen and Frank's wife showed me up the stairs into a spotlessly clean bedroom. She made a brief introduction and then left us.

Dear Lord, tell me what to say . . . let me be of some help to him . . .

I sat down on the edge of the bed.

'Hello, Frank, I hear we're in the same club?'

'Yes.' His fingers plucked restlessly at the sheets and he stared at me.

Eventually he said, 'You're doing a good job, aren't you? I don't know how you can be bothered when they've told you you've not long to live.'

'I'm not doing it alone, Frank. I'm getting an awful lot of help from an awful lot of people.'

'What's your trouble. Where is it?'

I told him.

'Mine's asbestosis. They've given me three months. I can't understand it. I handle very little of the stuff in my work. I don't know why I have to get this. It's so bloody unfair!'

'Life isn't always fair to us, is it, love?'

He studied my face, taking in my rosy complexion.

'There doesn't *look* much wrong with you, does there?' was his next comment.

There was a silence between us, and then:

'D'you believe in God?'

'Yes, Frank, I do.'

'D'you think there's a life after this life on earth?'

'I'm sure there is.'

'I don't. I don't believe that there's anything else when we die. That's it. Finish.'

Another silence.

'It's not easy, Frank. I'm not going to pretend that any of it is easy.'

'You're damned right it's not!' He fought to keep some measure of composure. 'How old are you?'

'Fifty', I replied. 'Time is a relative thing, Frank. When you think of all the millions of years this earth has been spinning round on its axis, we human beings are on it for a very short time. A human life is of very short span compared with all the time of eternity.'

'It doesn't make you feel any better about it, does it,' he replied.

'No, it doesn't, but look at it this way . . . you may not have very long and I may not have very long. What really matters is not *how long* we live, but what we do with the time we've got left. For instance, you're not in too much pain at the moment, are you?'

He shrugged his shoulders.

'I'm not so bad.'

'You love your wife and children don't you?'

'Of course I do!'

'Then why aren't you downstairs, sitting in a deck chair in the garden, watching your children at play and enjoying their company? What sort of memories are you going to leave them of YOU? It's a lovely day. Enjoy your family and enjoy the sunshine while you can. Make every day count – FOR THEM. It'll be time enough to stay in that bed when you become too ill to get out of it.'

'I suppose you're right,' he said reluctantly.

'I know I am! Come on, lad, keep fighting. Try putting a smile on your face – if not for yourself, then for that pretty wife of yours and those two lovely children.'

'I'll try.'

'That's the spirit. Don't try to face more than one day at a time, Frank. Tomorrow's not here, yet. Cope with that when it comes.'

'Yes, I see what you mean.'

'I'll go now, Frank. I mustn't tire you. Bless you and good luck.'

We shook hands.

'Same to you. Thanks for coming.'

I don't know how my legs carried me down the stairs.

In the kitchen, Mrs Frank offered me a cup of tea, but all I wanted was a drink of cold water. One of the girls dashed in from the garden to ask for a drink of orange cordial. She downed it in quick *slicks*, eager to get back to whatever game they were playing. As Mrs Frank rinsed the glasses, I said that I didn't know whether I'd done any good or not.

She smiled.

'Well anyway, thanks for trying. I appreciate it.'

As my friend and I drove away from the cottage, I felt drained.

Some weeks later, she rang to tell me that Frank had died.

'Oh dear . . . I suppose it was inevitable. How's his wife. How has she taken it?'

'She's not so bad. She's coping.'

'I wonder if that visit did any good?'

'Oh yes. She said he'd spent quite a lot of time in the garden on his good days, until he had to take to his bed. She said to let you know.'

The Tale of Two Rings is worth the telling . . .

From time to time, pieces of jewellery have been donated to the Fund. Usually, they have belonged to someone who has departed this life; the next of kin do not always wish to keep the pieces to wear themselves and some have chosen to donate them in memory of the person to whom they belonged. The stories behind the two rings did not fall into this category. They were given for such widely diverse reasons.

Early one evening, the phone rang. It was a lady who said she lived in a town some forty miles away. She had something rather valuable which she did not want to send to me by post – could she bring it for me that evening? I said it was rather a long way to come and asked what it was. She said it was a ring. I replied that if she'd feel happier delivering it by hand, it was fine by me. It was one of my rare nights at home and we arranged that she would arrive at about eight o'clock.

When Mrs A arrived, she took out of her handbag a small jeweller's box, opened it to display a most beautiful gold ring, set with three large, perfectly matched diamonds.

'I'd like you to have this for the Fund,' she said. 'And if you don't mind, I'd like to tell you why I'm giving it to you.'

It seemed Mrs A had a little grandson, a child she idolised. From being a lively, healthy little boy who was the light of Mrs A's existence, he had suddenly been taken ill and within a short time, his life was in danger. For days on end, there were no signs of improvement and his parents and his grandmother were distraught with worry. Mrs A realised that there wasn't one single thing she possessed that was as valuable to her as the life of her grandson. Looking at the ring, sparkling on her finger and which she had been nervously twisting like a worry bead, she vowed to herself, there and then, that if only the child could be well again, she would donate the ring to some worthy cause. Eventually, the boy's condition took a turn for the better. Steadily, he began to improve. After a period of convalescence, he eventually returned to his former state of good health. That was why Mrs A came to see me, to donate her token of thanksgiving. Eventually, the ring was sold for a three-figure sum and it is now worn by a charming young lady who was very moved to hear the story behind her new acquisition.

The second ring came by registered post. It was a woman's wedding ring. Without offering any reason, the gentleman who sent it merely wrote to say he wished to donate it to the Fund. I took it to a local jeweller, who said he could only offer the scrap gold value. Maybe the donor would expect it to be worth more than that? Pauline and I decided we had better consult him before disposing of it and duly wrote to him. A few days later, back came his reply. To say the least, it surprised us. We had imagined him to be a widower, but this was not the case. He said that the ring was of no sentimental value whatsoever; it had belonged to his wife, who had run off with another bloke. He said she had wanted a sugar daddy instead of a *man*. He never wanted to see that ring again and we could do what the hell we liked with it!

Of such facets the kaleidoscope of human nature is fashioned.

At many of the events I have attended I have been presented with bouquets or flower arrangements. They have given me a great deal of pleasure. There have been times when I have run out of flower vases and, though I am no expert at flower arranging, I do like fiddling about with flowers in an attempt to display them to best advantage, often using the result as the subject for one of my miniature flower paintings. Sometimes, when I just haven't had enough surfaces on which to put them all, I've given some to my mother, or to some elderly housebound person, someone just home from hospital or, if it's near to weekend, put them in church. At the Grand Theatre, Blackpool, in the spring of 1978, Manager Bob

Parsons said to his Saturday afternoon Bingo ladies: 'When you come next week, it will be the day before Mothering Sunday. It would be nice if we were to send Mrs Seed some flowers.'

Bless them, the next Saturday they brought flowers or flowering plants. Margaret Parkinson picked them up and brought them to Garstang for me. Their overwhelming kindness resulted in thirty-six bunches of daffodils, plus irises, narcissi, lilies, carnations, roses, African violets . . . I could have opened a florist's shop. Our home was filled with fragrance and colour and so was our parish church. All Things Bright and Beautiful . . . the following Saturday, I went to the Grand to thank the ladies, but I felt that anything I said was totally inadequate.

Beer and skittles? There have been plenty of nights like that, too. Enjoyable, rollicking nights in pubs and clubs, when somebody has played the piano, someone else has got up to sing a few songs, when good humour has flowed along with the ale and the spirits and the night has ended with the Fund several pounds better off.

I enjoy a drink myself, but drink and drugs don't mix. For me, it's usually one gin and tonic – and then for the remainder of the evening, it's just tonic or tomato juice.

But things aren't always bright and beautiful. There has been the other side of the coin.

Any charity is vulnerable to misuse. Most people are honest and straightforward, but, sadly, there is always the minority who will try to use some good cause for personal gain. This charity has not escaped entirely, although I think it has suffered less than one would expect.

There have been collecting boxes pinched off pub counters; this so upset one licensee that he and his customers organised a sponsored walk to make up the loss. They had estimated the box contained about £50, but their walk raised £600.

One chip-shop owner was so furious when our collecting

box was taken from his counter, that he considered putting a notice up, saying he hoped the thief got cancer. Then he thought better of it and organised a raffle to make good the loss. But I can understand how he felt.

When I hear of things like this, I am saddened. I am also angry. When so many people have put in so much time and effort to raise money and others have given at great personal sacrifice, I cannot but feel that such ill-gotten gains will never do the thieves any good. Such people will never prosper.

Whenever I have had any doubts, or when the branch committees have been doubtful about a set of circumstances, we have had no hesitation in asking the police to check for us. This, they have done. People have been cautioned, one person is serving a prison sentence and the affairs of another are still the subject of police investigation, involving endless, pains-taking sifting.

Many north-west Constabularies – and some from further afield – have made contributions to the Fund. Rochdale Police organised a sponsored walk in which thirty-two members of the force, together with office staff, took part, and one night in May 1978, in their Social Club, presented me with a four-figure cheque. One Lancashire constable, weighing twenty-two stones, went on a sponsored slim! Staines, Middlesex, Police sent their donation with the following verse:

> There was a young lady called Pat
> Who wanted to purchase a CAT
> That's the name of the scanner,
> So the cops in this manor
> Decided to pass round the hat.
> The helmet went on the rounds
> And we put in our pennies and pounds.
> We aint got a lot,
> But it's not what we got –
> It's the thought behind it that counts.

The thought behind it . . . no human being is entirely bad. From the other side of the law, I received a donation from a man serving a sentence in Liverpool's Walton Jail. The parcel arrived through the post and it is to the credit of The Post Office that this delicate piece of craftsmanship was undamaged, for Richard's contribution was an exquisite traditional gipsy caravan – made entirely out of matchsticks. On the tiny porch, was a rocking chair, two little dogs. carriage lamps either side of the door, a besom (a brush made of twigs) standing in the corner and even a bird in a cage, hanging from the porch roof. Inside, was a bed, a table on which Richard said were two pieces of prison bread which he didn't recommend anyone to eat! On the back wall were two tiny pictures of his children. A beautiful piece of work which must have taken him hours to make. Both sides of the law, helping the Fund. And why not? 'Big C' as it is often called does not differentiate between the law man and the law breaker.

You name it, people have done it in support of the Fund. Folks have thought up some weird, wonderful and ingenious ideas. Some of them have had me shaking with laughter, others have reduced me to tears and some have had me biting my nails, thankful when some exploit is over.

In the latter category are the intrepid individuals and groups of adventurous lads and lasses who have pitched themselves out of planes on the ends of parachutes – never having done so before! I couldn't do it, if my life depended upon it. When I've known these jumps were to take place, I've worried myself sick in case someone was hurt. Maybe it's a hangover from the war. As a girl, I remember being horrified by reports of the Arnhem landings and the terrible death toll which resulted. I remember thinking that these army parachutists must be just about the bravest soldiers on earth. Many were the target of snipers' bullets before they even reached the ground. I know that now parachuting is regarded as a sport and it has come a long way since those wartime days. I can appreciate that some find it an exhilarating experience, but much as I enjoy travelling by plane, I have that fatalist wartime approach to it! If a bomb's got your name on it, you'll cop it wherever you are. The thought of parachuting makes me shudder; it would never 'turn me on'. Be that as it may, I appreciate that some people find it almost addictive. I have the greatest admiration for their courage and there is no doubt that a considerable amount of money has been added to the Fund by this means. That also, I appreciate.

In complete contrast to those for whom the sky is the limit, there was a chap who wanted to bury himself alive, to beat the Guinness Book of Records (sponsored, of course). I am not sure what the outcome of that story was. The last I heard, nobody would lend him a piece of ground!

Then there was the streaker . . . Attending a charity night in a pub, the lady who was chairman of the local branch of the Appeal stood up, towards the end of the evening, to say a few words of thanks. She said that people were contributing in very many ways, doing their own thing, doing whatever they did best. A voice at one side of the bar piped up: 'I bet nobody has done a sponsored streak!' This rather threw the chairman. Somewhat embarrassed, she replied:

'Well, no. I don't think we've had one of those.'

'I'll do one for you,' said the voice.

Some wag at the back of the room shouted; 'I've got £7 here which says you won't!' To the consternation of my branch chairman, who found herself wishing she was a thousand miles away, the owner of the voice peeled off his clothes, ran round the pub, got dressed and then went to collect the £7.

'The things I do for this Fund!' said the chairman, as she told me all about it on the telephone the next day. 'It'll be a long time before I show my face in THAT pub again!'

'Never mind . . . as long as it's only your face you're showing, that's OK.'

A letter arrived one morning from two students at a local agricultural college. The students had enclosed their cheque and said that the money had been raised by a sponsored egg-eating session. One of them had eaten twenty-seven raw eggs in an hour and a quarter, sponsored by his friends. The letter was signed, Alistair (Sponsorship Secretary) and Martyn (egg-eater). *Twenty-seven raw eggs!* I rang the *Garstang Guardian*'s sub-editor. The following Friday, the front page carried a picture of Martyn swallowing a raw egg out of a glass, together with his story. 'It all started off as a joke, really,' he said. 'We were discussing the Paul Newman film *Cool Hand Luke* in which he had to eat eggs for a bet. That was when I decided to do it. I sat there with a waste paper basket handy, just in case I needed it, but fortunately, I didn't.'

Some weeks later another student at the college shaved off all his hair in support of the Fund. As this coincided with a really cold winter spell with frost and several inches of snow on the ground, his fellow students decreed that he should not wear a hat for three weeks. The last I heard was that he'd raised £70 so far. I daresay he's come in for a lot of ribald remarks from fellow students, but as he's a brawny six foot three, I should think twenty-year-old Andrew Midgley is quite capable of giving anyone who carries it too far, a sizable punch on the nose!

Talking about eggs, reminds me of a joke told by comedian Teddy Corvo at a Gala Charity Performance at Blackpool's Opera House.

He remarked on the different standard of 'digs' in which stage people stayed and said that during one Blackpool season, he and a fellow artiste had put up at a Fylde farmhouse. Whether this is factual or not, is irrelevant. In his deadpan Liverpool accent, he told us:

'There were about sixty chickens and one big fat pig – that didn't include the landlady . . .' (laughter). 'The first morning we had fried eggs for breakfast. The second morning, we had boiled eggs. On the third morning, we had scrambled eggs, but my pal said to me, "Hey, I think we might be getting a slice of bacon in the morning." I said to him, "Oh? What makes you think that?" He said, "Well, I've just looked out of the window. The pig's got an elastoplast on its bum!" '

Teddy was co-compère with Kenny Raye, chairman of the Gala committee who had arranged the Charity Performance. The huge theatre was packed, there was a starstudded cast, with artistes giving their performances for fees much below their normal rates. We raffled a football, donated by the Football Association and signed by the England team; a cathedral design, hand-made patchwork quilt, a beautiful piece of work donated by a lady from Harlow, Essex, and a painting of Haworth, Yorkshire given by the artist, David Oxley, OBE. This raffle raised £581 making the evening's grand total over £3,000 profit. It was on the stage of the Opera House on this night, that our Competition winners received their prizes – and thereby hangs another tale, again involving the law, this time in the form of the Lotteries Act. To hold an 'instant' type of raffle at a small event, within the confines of church or school hall or in someone's home, cloakroom tickets may be used and no licence is required. However, if tickets are to be sold to the general public for some weeks before being drawn, a licence from the local borough or city council is required. The raffle tickets must state where and when the draw is to take place and they must be numbered; they must also give the name and address of the promoter. On completion of this type of raffle, which comes under the Small Lotteries Act, a return must be sent to the local council who issued the licence. It must state the amount collected, plus any expenses deducted. These licences cost £10 renewable every January at £5. For a bigger raffle, with more valuable prizes, for which tickets are to be sold over a much wider area, one needs a licence from the Gaming Board of Great Britain.

I had been offered a car, five hundred poundsworth of furniture or carpets and a holiday for two in Malta. I telephoned the Gaming Board, to be told that the value of the main prize must not exceed £2,000.

'Who can buy a car for £2,000, these days?'

'Those are the rules,' said my informant.

'How on earth do these large firms – cornflakes manufacturers, for example – get away with it? They give prizes of much greater value than this – status-symbol cars and even houses?'

'Ah, that's different. In those cases, it isn't a raffle, it's a competition in which there is an element of skill. In that case, you don't need a licence from anyone.'

So *that*'s how it's done . . . So we'll make it a competition. John Wilding (Garstang) Ltd had donated a Ford Fiesta. John and two of his senior staff listed eight features of the Fiesta, to be put in order of merit. And if we were to have a slogan, I decided that in furtherance of the removal of the fear which surrounds the word Cancer, we would ask competitors to devise a slogan which they thought would encourage people to seek help in time.

Thus, the requirements of the law were met.

But nowadays when people have to fill in forms for just about everything, it did put a lot of people off buying the entry forms. The forms were distributed to the branches, whose members did their best to sell as many as possible. Some were more successful than others, but all of them agreed that, had they been raffle tickets, they'd have sold like the proverbial hot cakes. However, it did make over £3,500 for the Fund.

The slogans were judged by Mr Rennie Davison, Director of the Manchester Regional Committee for Cancer Education, and myself. We scrutinised thousands of entry forms, narrowing the field down to thirty-six, then twelve and then four. We then copied out on blank forms the features of the car and gave them to Mr Wilding, who did not know the names or addresses of the finalists. He and his staff devised a points system. The order of merit was 24, 21, 19 and 15 points – and so, we had our three winners, and as it happened they came from differing parts of the north-west.

The Brumgrove Club, Blackpool, had donated the holiday and on behalf of the Club, Mr and Mrs Ted Collinson presented the voucher to Mrs I. Williams of Wrexham, North Wales, whose slogan was 'While you're being frightened, you could be being cured'. Mr Leslie Whiston and his wife, of Talbot Road Salerooms, Blackpool, presented Mrs Susan Graves of Lancaster with a voucher for £500 of carpets or furniture of her choice. Mrs Graves' slogan was: 'Fear could be fatal, when the cancer could be cured'. The stage curtains were opened and there was a gleaming white Fiesta. Mr and Mrs John Wilding handed over the car keys to Mr Ray Lee of Lytham, whose slogan was 'Life – a test in time saved mine'.

All of these slogans are good and are now the copyright of the Regional Committee for Cancer Education. The winners were, of course, delighted with their prizes and the competition was only made possible by the generosity of the donors, to whom I offer my grateful thanks.

The staff of another firm sent me the contents of *their* office swear box, complete with the lid of the box, which listed the rules (non union). Sent from the 'Cost Office Lot – and Other Odds and Sods' the rules included winnings from cards, normal swear words – 1p; words used in lieu of – 1p; ten swear words, VAT to be paid – 11p; not swearing for a week – penalty 5p; paying in advance, two swear words for 1p. No credit given! Visitors only: non-optional voluntary payments!

There are all kinds of love . . .

Our Garstang Ladies Circle put on a Caribbean Night at our local village hall. The hall was decorated with fish nets, baubles, lanterns and the tables groaned with a colourful buffet of West Indian dishes. About ten thirty in the evening a West Indian Steel Band from Preston came on stage.

'Sorry they're late,' whispered Elizabeth, the President, as the strains of 'Yellow Bird' filled the room. 'They didn't finish on the late shift at Courtauld's factory until ten o'clock. They've come straight from work.' Then she added, 'They're giving their performance for free,' and, pointing to a young man on the left of the stage, added, 'That one's mother died of cancer only a month ago.'

I looked at the musicians, at the perspiration streaming down their dark faces as their melodious rhythmic tunes permeated the hall. My eyes filled with tears and, as unobtrusively as possible, I made my way outside. Elizabeth followed me.

'Oh, Elizabeth, what does it matter what colour our skins are? Cancer doesn't discriminate – why should we?'

Cancer has taught me many things. Among them is the fact that we human beings don't think big enough. Here we are, on one small planet, spinning endlessly through space using up energy arguing about territorial boundaries, becoming bitter, hostile and sometimes downright violent because the other chap's skin may be a different colour than ours. He may eat a different kind of food, worship a different God, wear different clothes, speak in a different tongue . . . yet we are all of us human, and all of us eligible for cancer. That young West Indian boy probably loved his mother every bit as much as I love mine. Here he was, doing the thing he did best to help raise money for a machine to help other cancer sufferers. We were harnessed to the same yoke and the colour of our skins was of no consequence whatsoever. This was the kind of incident which could only renew my determination. I'd see that scanner installed at the Christie, or die in the attempt. It could be one or the other. Time would sort that out. Meanwhile, there was work to be done. I'd use every ounce of energy I possessed in pursuit of the objective, knowing that there were plenty of good people to help me along the way.

'Do you feel like a night out?'

'Why, where are you heading for this time?'

'Not so far away tonight. I'm going to a Labour Club near Preston.'

'In that case, we shouldn't get lost, should we?'

At about eight thirty Marie and I arrived at the Larches Club at Lea. The large clubroom was already crowded and, on stage, three young men were playing guitars and singing songs.

The officials of the club welcomed us and then escorted us to a table at the front and to the left of the stage.

On the table was a card on which were the words: 'Reserved for Artists'.

I nudged Marie.

'What are you going to do?'

She gave me a filthy look.

On the right-hand side of the table, sat an extremely attractive, dark-haired young lady and her boy friend. On the other side, were two tiny, small-boned bird-like women. They were identical twins whose age would be somewhere around the sixty mark.

We all exchanged greetings and made polite conversation. I kept looking at the 'Reserved for Artists' and then at the twins and I just could not imagine what their act might be, or how they were going to entertain us. Maybe those two seats just happened to be vacant . . . Eventually, the young lady and her boy friend got up and went behind the stage. The trio of guitarists made their final bow to enthusiastic applause. Having changed into a ravishing evening dress, the brunette sang four songs, concluding with 'Don't cry for me, Argentina'. She had an excellent voice, a good stage presence and was an accomplished artiste.

Between songs, curiosity got the better of me. I asked the twins, 'Are you artistes?'

'Oh yes,' they said, without the ghost of a smile, 'we're a comedy act.'

As our conversation until then had consisted mostly of putting the world to rights, the price of food and the previous Sunday's scandal in the *News of the World*, we had certainly seen no evidence of comedy so far.

Solemnly, one of them informed us, 'We're the Nutters.'

'Oh,' I said, even more mystified.

Next came the interval, during which the raffle was drawn. There were endless prizes and it seemed as though there were almost as many as there were people in the room, demonstrating yet again the good-hearted generosity of folk who were backing the Appeal to the hilt. Then the Club Chairman reminded everyone what the purpose of the evening was and he presented me with a substantial cheque. There was a super atmosphere in the club, again typical of many such occasions I'd seen along the 'Scanner Trail'. I said a few words of thanks to the committee, the members and their guests and then, when I rejoined Marie, the twins had disappeared, somewhere backstage.

'What d'you suppose they do?' asked Marie, but before I could think of an answer, the Club Secretary came staggering across the room with a gallon whisky bottle in his arms. It was full to the brim with coppers. He banged it down on the table in front of us and said:

'Here! We're not counting that bloody lot – take it home with you!'

'Take it home with me? I couldn't even lift it!'

'Don't worry, love, we'll put it in your car for you when you leave.'

As I tried to thank him, the stage curtains swished back to reveal the twins – in Carmen Miranda outfits, complete with huge baskets of fruit on their heads. And along with the costumes, they'd donned competely new personalities. Vivaciously, and in intentionally flat Lancashire accents, they sang 'I,I,I,I,I,I love you verr-ry much . . .' They'd hardly got to the third 'I' when the audience were in stitches and Marie nearly disappeared under the table. When one of their frilly skirts fell off, there was an uproar. There followed another Latin American song, the title of which I cannot remember. It was sung in Spanish, and with an accent no Spaniard worthy of his salt would own.

By this time, our ribs were aching and Marie and I along with a lot of others in the audience, were dabbing at our eyes with our handkerchiefs. But the Nutters hadn't finished with us yet. The organist started to play 'The Stripper' music; the twins disappeared from our view to the back of the stage, which we could not see from where we were sitting. They reappeared at the front of the stage, dressed in black tights, red bloomers and short, white satin mini-dresses.

'Keep your hand on your Ha'penny, Mary,' they sang – and they did!

It's one thing to laugh politely. It's quite another to roll in the aisles, especially when you're the guests of honour. By this time, neither Marie nor I could speak. We were helpless. Trying to keep a grip on myself, I looked at my watch. 'Come on – it's turned eleven. We'd better go before we disgrace ourselves.'

Some things are meant to be funny and some are not. It's when something amuses you at non-humorous events that things get difficult or downright embarrassing. There have been occasions like this, when it's taken all my self-control to keep a straight face.

My mother and I had visited friends in the Manchester area, making an afternoon of it and having tea with my friend of over forty years, Mrs Beryl Acton. That night, I'd to attend a presentation at a Bingo hall near to where Beryl lives and she, knowing my aptitude for getting lost, drove us there in her car.

When we got there, the vast room was filled with, I should guess, about 1,000 people, all busily marking off numbers on cards as they were intoned by the caller or appeared on strategically placed, closed circuit TV screens. Beryl and I were talking to the ladies who had held several fund-raising efforts over a period of time which had resulted in the cheque they were to present to me.

'We'll just get this round of games over with and then we'll have a break and make the presentation,' they whispered to me.

Apart from the caller's voice, the silence was such that it would have made the morgue seem like the palace of varieties. My little mother knows nothing about Bingo. She'd sat down on a chair a few yards away next to a man who was marking several cards. In her usual fashion, she was keeping in the background and leaving me to it. Mother tried to engage the man in conversation. He was concentrating on numbers. The organisers were trying to tell Beryl and me, in undertones, how the money had been raised. I could hear my mother's voice, saying what a big place it was and what a lot of people, etc.

'Do they come here every night?' she asked, in her normal speaking voice.

'Bloody hell, I missed that one, then! Shut up, will you!'

My mother's face was a study. It registered astonishment and disbelief. I laughed out loud and it was a wonder all three of us weren't thrown out. In a way, we were. We were hurriedly shepherded into a sound-proofed office where the rules – written and unwritten – were explained to Mum. She had not realised that substantial sums of money were at stake and that some folk regard Bingo more as a religion than a game.

The Tax Man cometh ... missives from the income tax office usually put your heart in your boots, but one I received from the staff of HM Inspector of Taxes office at Barrow-in-Furness held no fears or portents of disaster.

In aid of the Fund, they had arranged a whole series of events, which denoted their originality and imagination and which took place over a number of weeks. The entire staff took part and they had plenty of fun in the process. Letters, keeping me informed of their activities, suggested that the Tax Inspector just had to have a sense of humour to keep pace with them. The only time he 'drew the line' was when they'd arranged a Karate Exhibition and wanted to use him as the demonstration model! My friend Hazel Woodward and I drove to Barrow one night to attend one of their fund-raising evenings and as their letters suggested, they were a real jolly crowd. Also there, were our friends from the Barrow Soroptimists and it was good to meet them again. If the truth were told, we didn't really need a branch of the Fund in Barrow. The Soroptimists had assumed the role, acting as agents for me and their staunch support during the entire Appeal has resulted in several thousands of pounds added to the Fund. The trip to Barrow-in-Furness also meant that I had now visited each of the furthermost places of the area served by the Christie – Barrow, Kendal, Crewe and Wrexham. People, people, people, and the common denominator was kindness. That night in Barrow was typical of what was happening all over the north-west.

'I wonder what's happened to our pensioner this week?' I said to Pauline, 'I hope she's all right.'

Over several months, on either Friday or Saturday of each week, there is a familiar envelope among the mail. It's addressed to Pat Seed, 'THE CANCER WOMAN', Garstang, Lancs. Inside, there is a folded scrap of paper on which is written: 'May you live for ever and ever. For years and years. God bless you – A Pensioner.' Wrapped in the paper are just a few coppers. Sometimes there's 15p, 19p, 23p and one week, 30p.

I would think that when this pensioner goes to the post office each week to collect her money, she sends to me whatever she has left out of the previous week's pension.

This particular week, it didn't arrive. I wondered if she was ill (why did I assume the sender was a woman?) and in need of help. I felt quite worried about her. She is one of the many unseen, unknown friends the Appeal has brought me. I'd grown fond of my pensioner. The following week, her small change was accompanied by a note: 'Sorry we couldn't send you anything last week. It was our fiftieth anniversary and we had to buy a cake and have it iced for our golden wedding, so we were a bit short.'

Maybe the reader will appreciate what I mean when I say you need nerves of steel to do this job and what it is that drives me on and renews my incentive.

I would like to gather that dear old couple in my arms and give them a hug – and then take them out for a slap-up meal. But there is never a name, never an address. The only clues are that the coppers are sometimes wrapped in a *Manchester Evening News* classified ads form and the postmark, when it is decipherable, is Manchester.

On a visit to friends in Florida, USA, a Lancaster farmer, Bill Sutcliffe, happened to be watching his host's television set one evening. The film being screened showed a charity concert, filmed in Hawaii, and starred the late Elvis Presley. As Bill watched the film, ideas began to flow and when he returned home to his farm at Cockerham, south of Lancaster, he began to put them into practice. As his own father had died of cancer, Bill identified with the Appeal. Anything he could do to help, he would do. And he's not the sort of chap who does things by halves.

For many years, he and a group of his friends were known as the Silver Keynotes Band. They'd played in just about every dance hall within a radius of twenty miles. Fine musicians, they'd enjoyed a lot of popularity and had quite a following. About five or six years ago, as other interests took over, the musicians had disbanded.

However, ringing around his friends and putting his idea to them, the band got together again for just one special occasion, in aid of the Fund, the Lancaster and District Farmers' Ball in Lancaster's Ashton Hall. The tickets were a sell out before they were even printed and they could have been sold three times over. As it was, on the night of the dance almost 1,000 people packed into the Ashton Hall and for many of the dancers, it was a nostalgic trip down memory lane. Married couples, who now had growing families, relived their courting days as they danced to the Silver Keynotes Band. Many who had not met each other for years renewed friendships and caught up on recent news of acquaintances, many tried to persuade the band to re-form. The evening raised £2,000 for the Fund and everyone had a memorable time.

But that wasn't the end of it, or Bill's only idea. For the farming community, artificial insemination of cattle is a commonplace modern method of improving the quantity and quality of stock. A measure of AI is known as a 'straw'. Owners of pedigree Friesian bulls had donated some twenty 'straws' to be used as raffle prizes at the dance, but as plenty of other prizes had been donated, Bill decided these offerings could be used to better advantage as a separate raffle. He organised the AI semen draw as another effort and tickets were sold to farmers in many parts of England, Scotland and Wales. As these raffle tickets circulated, I came in for some ribbing and one journalist friend shrieked with laughter down the telephone, saying, 'My God, Pat, you'll put your name to anything!'

OK – it may be somewhat amusing, yet nobody thinks twice about buying the produce of these animals – butter, milk or cream – at bring-and-buy events. In various parts of Britain, there are now animals, young heifers and bull calves, who arrived in this world as donations to the Appeal Fund. What is more, they have added yet another £2,000 to it.

Following the dance, Bill and his sister Marion – both of them are talented vocalists – decided to cut a record and made a single recording which sold like hot cakes and added another £250 to the coffers. Bill now has thoughts about an LP of the Silver Keynotes. At the time of writing, he's off on an agricultural study tour of San Francisco, New Zealand, Australia and Singapore, I'm wondering what ideas he'll bring back with him this time . . .

There's no people like show people . . . and those I've met on the 'Scanner Trail' have been big-hearted folk. For their Derby Day at Blackpool Greyhound Stadium in 1977 the management invited stars who were appearing on stage in the town's theatres during the summer holiday season, to come along and sign their autographs at 20p a time for the Fund. This was how I came to meet Eric Sykes, Hattie Jacques and Derek Guyler; Little and Large, Frank Carson, the Black Abbots. The following year, Marti Caine, Paul Daniels and Colin Crompton came along and did the same thing.

When you are appearing twice nightly for six nights a week during Blackpool's minimum sixteen-week season (and the famous Illuminations can extend this to twenty-two weeks) life can get very exhausting. And when you don't get to bed until the small hours of the morning, it is something of a sacrifice to turn up, bright and cheerful, at 11 a.m. Hattie Jacques told me, 'One tries to hold something back for the second performance each night, but you find yourself giving it all you've got at both performances – that's what the audience have paid for.'

'What are you going to do when the season ends? Take a holiday or just go home and put your feet up for a while?'

'Go home and put my feet up. That's as good as a holiday in this profession.'

In the wings of Blackpool's Grand Theatre when he appeared in the Super Star Night, Colin Crompton told Geoff (I was on stage at the time): 'Pat Seed! I've nearly killed myself for Pat Seed.'

Somewhat startled, Geoff had asked, 'Why? What happened?'

'I took part in one of these charity cricket matches for the Fund. I'm still aching in every limb and I've not got over it yet!'

And then I came off stage and he said, 'Hello Pat. I'm Colin Crompton.'

Geoff said to me later, 'Now I've heard everything – it should have been the other way round!'

Television names have done an awful lot to help me. Bob Smithies, Granada's Reports newscaster and reporter, has interviewed me for the programme and has also opened garden fêtes and fairs for the Fund. Stuart Hall, presenter of BBC's 'Look North' programme and who commentates the international 'It's a Knock Out' programme, has a sadly depleted wardrobe. When I met him at an event in Preston Guild Hall, he greeted me with:

'Pat Seed! I've given away ties, socks, shirts, pullovers, a jacket and even a pair of trousers for that Fund of yours!'

I grinned. 'Never mind – you could always do a streak.'

'You'd get me run in!' he replied in mock horror.

The occasion happened to include a cookery demonstration using microwave cookers. Stuart, wearing striped apron and straw hat, was ably assisting the lady demonstrator with an ad lib commentary. Also there was comedian Les Dawson.

When the demo had got as far as a beef stroganoff flambé, Stuart decided it was time Les did a bit of work and invited him to flame the dish. But after Les had doused about seven matches in the stroganoff, they gave him up as a bad job. If the flambé was a damp squib, the repartee between Stuart and Les was a huge success with the audience.

The cast of Granada's most famous programme 'Coronation Street' which is supposedly based in my home town of Salford, has top audience rating in Britain and is popular in many Commonwealth countries. Practically all the cast of this programme have done their stint for the Fund. They've made personal appearances, opened garden parties, attended many north-west night clubs, opened flower shows; when a national weekly paper did a series of articles about Julie Goodyear (barmaid Beth) she waived her fee in favour of the Fund. At Manchester's Golden Garter night club, Rolf Harris, Australia's international star, topped the bill at a charity night jointly sponsored by the club and by the *Manchester Evening News*. He donated one of his 'instant paintings' to be auctioned – profits for the Fund.

Geoff and I spent a memorable evening 'According to Kossoff' when Grange Round Table invited him to give his performance in a local hall as a money-raising effort. Later, Tabler Fred Nixon and his wife Elaine invited us all back to supper. David Kossoff is not only a top flight actor and writer, he's a very kindly person and an excellent raconteur. We discussed life and religion in all aspects until the small hours of the morning. As we left, David put his hands on my shoulders, looked into my eyes and kissed me on the forehead with the word 'Shalom' being the Jewish word for Peace. I knew he meant it as a blessing.

It is impossible to mention all the names of the show business stars and TV personalities who have helped or all the acts, large and small, who have stood up on stages and entertained in support of the Fund. They are a truly great breed of people and I am eternally grateful to them all.

11

Some Peaks and a Trough

As I said before, time after time I have been taken aback by
some of the things that have happened and have been left
wondering what else could possibly happen to surprise me.
August 1978 and life hadn't finished surprising me yet. A
letter arrived inviting me to attend The Women of the Year
Luncheon at the Savoy Hotel, London, in September — as a
guest of honour!

Who? Me? My first thought was that somebody had
slipped up, got it all wrong. I read the letter, signed by Lady
Georgina Coleridge, three times before I took in its contents.

The Women of the Year Luncheon is an annual event in
aid of the Greater London Fund for the Blind to which
famous and noteworthy women are invited. As well as
raising several thousand pounds each year for this charity,
the Luncheon is a prestigious event in its own right. To be
asked to it is an accolade. To be asked to attend as one of the
guests of honour is even more so. Her Majesty Queen Elizabeth the Queen Mother is Patron and the luncheon is usually
attended by a lady of the Royal Family if Her Majesty is
herself unable to be present. Famous women from all walks
of life attend and it is probably the only occasion when so

many are gathered together in the same place at the same time. Every woman present would be at, or near the top of her particular tree, each one a success in her chosen profession, vocation or calling.

Why had I been asked? Oh, I know I'd founded a charity and was working hard, but then, so were lots of other people who were supporting the Pat Seed Appeal Fund. As far as I was concerned, Pat Seed was just an ordinary housewife and Mum. There was nothing extraordinary or special about Pat Seed.

Would I be expected to make a speech? What would I find to talk about that could be of interest to other guests? And oh, heavens, what does one wear for lunch at the *Savoy*? The more I thought about it, the more I got cold feet, and the more exasperated Geoff became.

'For goodness' sake, either accept the invitation and go and enjoy it, or write to say you can't attend and then forget the whole thing. If you are going to worry yourself to a frazzle like you did over going to the Palace, you'd be far better staying at home!'

And yet I wanted to go. How could I find out what it entailed? I rang my friend Marie Drury, a *Gazette* journalist who'd stood in for me when I'd already been committed to attend other events. 'Marie, d'you think you could find out for me just what is expected of me? I really don't know what I'm in for, what I'm expected to do, what I ought to wear or anything. I feel a complete ignoramus and I can't very well ring to ask these things myself.'

'Sure,' said Marie, 'we'll need to know some of those answers for the paper, anyway.'

Later in the day, Marie rang back.

'You can stop worrying. For a start, you won't be expected to make a speech. There'll be about 600 women there and about forty of you are guests of honour on the top table. As for clothes, you'll find that they wear anything from trouser suits, to sweater dresses, to quite elaborate creations – so the choice is yours. All that's expected of you is that you go along and enjoy it. Just think of all the interesting people you will meet.'

Feeling relieved and much happier about it, I began to look forward to it. It would be a completely new experience for me and yes, I *would* meet some interesting people. And there was no need to wonder what I would talk about. It was a good opportunity to listen, for all of those women at the luncheon would have done things worthy of note. It could be fascinating. The only decision left was, *what to wear*?

A lot of women are hoarders and the things we hoard are diverse. My weaknesses are books and dress materials. I hadn't had the luxury of sitting down to read a book for months, but I did have a cupboard full of dress lengths, and I found a length of light navy silk and some matching lace. The material and lace had cost me a fiver a year or more ago. I made it up in the current fashion; a loose style, gathered into a small yoke and appliqued the lace onto the skirt and the full sleeves, livening it up with a sparse scattering of seed pearls. I bought a hat which is nothing more than an alice band covered in navy petals, and stitched a few pearls to that.

I tried the outfit on and asked the family what it looked like. Nobody in this household could get big headed. The rest would cut them down to size in no uncertain terms. My son said, 'It's not bad,' which is the highest accolade he gives anything, including my cooking, so I felt reassured. My daughter, home on a visit, said it was fine and Geoff said it was 'very nice' before he disappeared behind his newspaper again. Praise indeed. If it had been a total disaster, the lot of them would have said so, without any hesitation. It was put in the wardrobe, ready for 'The Day'.

I never use my sewing machine without memory taking me back across the years to my Great Aunt Emma. She was a little grey wisp of a woman whose neat black dress was always covered with a starched white apron. She was a tailoress and the downstairs front parlour was her workroom. From the window, she kept a watchful eye on the neighbourhood as her busy fingers plied her needle. As a small girl I often visited her and more often than not, was press-ganged into picking up pins from underneath the workroom table. 'Your back is younger than mine!' she would say. The pins were enmeshed in the flotsam and jetsam of previous sewing jobs, remnants and scraps which to a small girl were like the treasures in Aladdin's Cave.

As well as pins, I searched for suitable silks, chiffons and bits of lace to add another creation to my dolls' wardrobes. Later, and if she happened to be in an especially affable mood, I was allowed to try out my skill, or, as is more likely, the lack of it, on the sewing machine. My feet were hardly able to reach the treadle and the resultant seams were about as straight as a river's route to the sea. Givenchy couldn't have been more pleased than I was with the result of my labours. The pressing of garments was achieved with the help of two flat irons, alternating between the table and the hob of her cheerful fire. To a small girl, they seemed to be of enormous weight and I remember that I needed two hands to lift one. The triangular scorch marks on the white sheeting cover were a testimony to the number of times the irons had been too hot.

Great Aunt Emma and I shared a predilection for Brazil nuts. To watch her wield a flat iron on them was a source of fascination to me and the perfect demonstration of the proverbial sledgehammer to crack a nut. Despite her diminutive size, she packed enough punch to floor Mohammed Ali and the nuts almost disintegrated under the onslaught. I was delighted when by some miraculous chance, one remained whole. Another flat iron was used to prop open the workroom door on warm days. This was essential, for even with the temperatures in the seventies, a fire was necessary to heat those irons.

A wedge-shaped section was missing from that workroom table. When electric irons had first come onto the market, Great Aunt Emma had bought one. Inadvertently left face down and switched on, the non-thermostatic gadget had burnt its way through two inches of solid wood before falling to the floor among all those pins and scraps of material.

I do not remember having been told who sorted out that particular chaos – perhaps it was the fire brigade – but that hole remained until Great Aunt Emma hung up her tape measure and she and the table retired.

By that time, I would be about seventeen and I inherited the sewing machine. It needed a Samson to lift or move it. It was an ancient Singer trade model, a 31K15. Robust and reliable, I think it would have sewed concrete. This vintage model has gone and my current sewing machine seems to do everything except play the National Anthem. I wish I had one of her flat irons, just as a keepsake, for they pulverised many a pound of Brazil nuts over the years. However, I do have my Great Aunt Emma's magnet, still as effective as ever after the better part of a century, for my mother, who is now seventy-eight, tells me that as a little girl, she was detailed to pick up pins, too.

Whether she realised it or not, my Great Aunt Emma left me a legacy. She has saved me many a pound by passing on to me some of her dressmaking skills and that ancient sewing machine, for I began young enough to find it a novelty. And as I grew older, a money saver. 'Here, tack along that seam for me, or the devil will find work for those idle fingers!' The old girl could be the very devil of a taskmaster, but I've had reason to be grateful for it.

The 'Scanner Trail' continued, with its work, its worry, and the usual mixture of sadness and laughter. There were journeys to Wrexham, Glossop, Stockport and Crewe, and to other places too. And always, there were the letters, but with Pauline to help, the administration workload was much easier. The latter part of August and the beginning of September was a comparatively quiet period, with many people taking their annual holiday. I made use of the unaccustomed lull in activities to get down to some household chores and visit friends I hadn't seen much of in recent months. Then in the middle of September, the pace hotted up again and things started to happen. As usual, it began with a phone call . . . Pauline, only moments before the phone rang, had commented that things were slack.

'Look, maybe you don't need me any more. There's no point in keeping me on if there isn't enough for me to do.'

'You never know, Pauline. Things are usually so hectic, we're chasing our own tails. At least the respite gives us time to catch up on filing and things like that. Be thankful. That phone could ring and we'd be as busy as ever. The Appeal's far from over yet.'

On the line was Bill Kerr Elliott, a reporter for BBC 'Nationwide' TV. They were considering doing a feature about the Appeal. Could producer Ian Taylor and he come to see me?

'You know "Look North" have covered the Appeal, don't you?'

'Yes, we know, but we think it could be interesting enough for national coverage. How d'you feel about it?'

'This Appeal has survived on publicity. I'll be extremely grateful for any help you can give. Thank you very much.'

I reported the conversation to Pauline, adding, 'What was that you were saying about giving in your notice?'

Remembering the Russell Harty Show, she said, 'Oh, my goodness – here we go again!' and then, 'It's uncanny. You were just saying the phone could ring and we'd find ourselves as busy as ever – you'd hardly got the words out of your mouth and it DID ring. This job's full of coincidences like that, isn't it?'

'I know. It happens time and time again. Anyway, make

the most of the slack period, while you can.'

Some days later, Ian and Bill arrived.

'How much do you know about this Appeal?' I asked them.

'Not a great deal,' they said.

I gave them an article I'd written for the *Manchester Evening News* and one Robin Thornber had written for *The Guardian*. 'Here – have a read. I'm just taking my mother home and then we'll fill in the details when I come back. I'll only be five minutes. Help yourselves to more tea and biscuits.'

As my parents live quite close to us, I was back in the house again before they'd finished reading. Then we discussed the Appeal, from its inception to the present time and Ian and Bill discussed what would be good for filming.

'What are you doing in the next week or so?'

I told them and added, 'If you could show just what this scanner does, I'd be grateful. So many people have given to this Fund without really knowing exactly what they are giving their money for. It worries me.' They did. They filmed the pictures produced by the scanner at the Manchester University Medical School and compared them with ordinary X-ray pictures. At the Christie, they filmed Doctor Todd who explained the spread of breast cancer and how curable it can be if caught in the early stages. For a week or more, I seemed to go everywhere with the 'Nationwide' film crew in tow, but the result was the most comprehensive TV coverage yet, in that it was not just me talking; it showed, so that viewers could see for themselves, many facets of the Appeal. It is amazing how much can be packed into a twelve-minute feature.

The opening sequence was filmed at the Grundy House Museum, Blackpool, where Elizabeth Wood, the well-known portrait painter, is the Curator. After the Russell Harty interview had been screened by Granada in July, Elizabeth had written to ask me if she could paint my portrait as her contribution to the Fund. She wanted to paint me wearing that red dress. She thought it was symbolic. I remarked, 'Funny you should say that. It's how I feel about it, too.'

'It's such a warm colour. It seems to represent all the warmth the Appeal has generated.'

'There's just one thing, Elizabeth. Don't make me look twenty-five, will you? I'm fifty!'

'If I made you look twenty-five, I'd miss twenty-five years experience out of the portrait,' she replied.

I sat for her on several occasions and at other times, Elizabeth worked from photographs. When the picture was nearly completed, she invited Geoff and me to go and see it. It was me. Just as I am. It neither overstated nor understated. There is an honesty about Elizabeth's work. The portrait had been painted for love and posterity, for it is destined to hang in the new department at the Christie when it is finished. It's a peculiar feeling to look at a portrait of yourself. It's rather uncanny and in a way, creepy. The thought crossed my mind that I'd never be dead as long as that portrait existed.

Geoff was delighted with it and said he wished he could have it.

'Look at that tilt of the head – that's just your mannerism. And look at those hands – I'd recognise them anywhere.'

'Well, you can't have it. It's not yours. Anyway, where on earth would you find space for a gallery size picture, five feet by four feet?' I asked him, trying to imagine it in our sitting room, which is twenty feet long. He has had to be content with some photographs of it, but photographs can never do justice to the craft of any artist, any more than prints of Constable or Turner paintings compare with the originals. And as the Nationwide crew filmed, using their high-powered lighting, the light bounced off the oil paint, making the dress look pink. Sitting next to the portrait, wearing the dress, the fabric absorbed the light, making it seem an even brighter shade of red.

The Women of the Year Luncheon was held on Monday,

25th September. Roy lent Geoff and me the London flat and we travelled down on the previous Friday, so that we could meet some Canadian friends who had returned to London after their holiday in Greece. Noel and Geoff had been the aircrew of a Mosquito in the RAF. Shared wartime experiences in the Middle East and Italy had forged a lifelong friendship between the two men and a regular exchange of letters is enlivened by the Canadians' periodic visits to England. Kay, Noel's wife, and I often wonder how the pair of them managed to squeeze into the confined quarters of a Mossie's cockpit, as both are over six feet tall. I know that when they arrived in the Middle East, Noel had flung their gas masks and capes on to the back of a passing lorry with 'I guess we won't need those things out here.' We had a lovely time with them until they caught a plane back to Vancouver on Sunday afternoon.

The following morning the Nationwide crew took some film of me putting on my hat and then, when I arrived at the Savoy, took film of me stepping out of the taxi. In the editing, both sequences were discarded. However, they did include some film of the reception, and of me talking to actress Molly Sugden who was one of the five speakers at the luncheon.

I met and talked with Lady Georgina Coleridge, Lady Penn, the Luncheon Committee Chairman, and with Lady Wilson, wife of the former Prime Minister. The 600 or so guests included women whose names were household words. Actresses Penelope Keith, Una Stubbs, Dulcie Gray, Gayle Hunnicut; TV personality Katie Boyle; Erin Pizzey, who has done much to help battered wives; Lady Bull, Governor of Holloway Prison; Dr Josephina de Vasconcellos, the sculptress.

As a journalist, I knew that practically every woman in the room was worthy of an interview and a write-up. But this was neither the time nor the place. It was like being shown a magnificent banquet, to be told you could only look – you couldn't eat. I found myself standing next to Victoria Holt. I said that I'd been reading one of her books in Roy's flat the night before and how much I'd enjoyed it.

'You must have travelled extensively to write with such authenticity of detail?'

She said she'd travelled around the world at least ten times. As one who was trying to make the transition from journalist to author, I asked Victoria what her working routine was. She said she was at her desk at seven thirty each morning and worked through until midday. My heart sank into my blue strap sandals. As one who is hardly *compos mentis* before eight thirty and not fit to be spoken to before ten o'clock, that routine wasn't for me. Later, Monica Dickens told me her routine began at *six* in the morning, that she scribbled away for a couple of hours with pen and pad and then went to feed her horses and her dogs. Later in the day she would read over her 'scribble', knock it into shape and type it. Apart from the six a.m. bit, that sounded more like me. But this conversation was some weeks later, when I had dinner with Monica and her charming husband, Commander Roy Stratton, in Manchester.

The luncheon was served in the blue and white Lancaster room at the Savoy. Her Royal Highness the Duchess of Kent was the principal guest of honour. Opposite me, on Monica's left, was Jacqueline du Pré. On my right, the Editor of BBC Woman's Hour, Miss Wyn Knowles and on my left a young lady, Miss Jane Pugh, who is the Duchess's Lady in Waiting. In the middle of the lunch Miss Pugh told me: 'The Duchess of Kent has especially asked to meet you. She is very interested in what you are doing. When this is over, I will make my way to that door (indicating a door on the right of the room). If you will come with me, please, the Duchess would like to speak to you when she has said her goodbyes.'

That was when I knocked over what was left of my glass of

wine and hoped that nobody noticed. If they did, they were too kind or too good mannered to comment.

The five speakers were Miss Jane Reed, Editor of *Woman's Own* magazine; Naomi James, the first woman to sail round the world alone and in record time; Dr Anne Birchall, Keeper of Greek and Roman Antiquities at the British Museum; Her Honour Judge Deborah Rowlands and Miss Molly Sugden. The theme was 'Survival' and each speaker drew on her own experiences for the content of her speech. With such widely differing experiences upon which to draw, the speeches provided interesting contrasts on the art of survival. Then suddenly, it was all over and the time was a quarter to three. It had started at eleven thirty and the time had flown.

In the passage beyond the Lancaster Room, we waited for the Duchess to take leave of our hostesses. As she came through the door, I hardly had time to curtsy, or say 'good afternoon, Ma'am', before she took my hand and asked me about the work I was doing, the scanner, the Christie and how many CAT machines there were in Britain. 'I'd like to help you. You must let me know if there is anything I can do.'

I felt morally obliged to tell her that there was more than one scanner appeal in the country, including one in her native Yorkshire.

'Oh? Who's running that?'

'There's a committee, Ma'am, but I'm afraid I don't know the names of the officials.' More questions followed, then finally:

'Now don't forget, if there's anything at all I can do to help you, please do let me know.'

I tried – inadequately – to express my appreciation for her kindness and interest, but before I could convey my gratitude to her, she was gone and I was standing alone in the passage, wondering if it had really happened. I sat down on a chair and for some reason my mind went back to the day the 'Look North' team had come to the Christie to interview Dr Todd and me. Just eighteen months ago, and nobody except me seemed to have any faith in the Appeal – either inside the Christie or outside of it – in those early days. It had come a long way since then. And now a member of our Royal Family had offered her help.

Back at the flat, I came down to earth and asked Geoff what he had been doing all day. After leaving me outside the Savoy he'd walked along the Embankment, revisited the Abbey, St Paul's Cathedral and then taken a look at Westminster Cathedral. Somewhere en route, he'd had a pub lunch. We burst out laughing. There's a heck of a lot of difference between lunching at the Savoy and having a pie and a pint in a pub! What is more, his feet were killing him after all that walking.

We travelled home on Tuesday and on my desk was a pile of letters which Pauline had left, ready for me to sign; there were several queries and a list of telephone messages. I came down to earth yet again.

That week, Nationwide completed their feature. They filmed a Market Fair arranged by the staff and children of St Thomas's School, Garstang, which I attended. When it was screened, every child in the school said they had seen themselves on television! They filmed my pigeon hole at the Sorting Office and the Nat-West's computer producing a print-out of the Fund total. On Wednesday night, I went to a Ladies Circle meeting at Poynton, south of Manchester, and on Friday evening to an event at the Jolly Roger pub in Fleetwood. Life had resumed its normal pace and the delights of London might never have been . . .

The programme was televised on Monday, 2nd October. By the 4th, mail was arriving from all parts of the country, in spite of the fact that in accordance with BBC policy, no address had been given. That week, I'd five days of engagements, plus a meeting of the Central Committee.

'I thought you were only supposed to do three a week,' said Pauline as I put on my coat, one morning.

'You know what thought did, don't you?'

'Yes – and it won't be a wedding you're going to, if you don't do as you are told. It'll be a funeral – your own!'

But as I drove along the motorway, I reflected on what she'd said. I knew she was right. I had that 'one degree under' feeling. It was nothing I could put my finger on, nothing tangible, no definite pain, just a feeling of unease, around my ribs. *Oh, forget it and get on with the job – you're imagining things!* I tried to shrug it off, but it didn't seem to work. As I looked at my diary for the rest of October and November – five days of each week were filled with engagements and some dates had three events in one day – I just didn't know how I was going to fulfil them all, or where I was going to find the strength. Yet, peering at my reflection in the mirror, I looked just about the healthiest specimen in the north-west.

Early in November, Tom Scott, editor of the *Lancaster Guardian* telephoned. When Tom rings, it's usually to ask me to cover some event for the paper. After an exchange of pleasantries, I waited to *hear* what he'd got lined up for me.

'By the way, you're our Citizen of the Year.'

'Am I? Good Lord!'

For the past ten years, the paper has invited readers to nominate the name of a person in the locality whom they consider eligible for this honour. Although the *Lancaster Guardian* series prints six editions each week, one of which is the *Garstang Guardian*, I'd always assumed that the Citizen of the Year Award was confined to the Lancaster district. I said as much to Tom.

'Oh no. It covers the whole circulation area. We'll have to arrange a presentation. When do you think you could manage it?'

'Not until December, Tom. I've hardly a free day this month.'

'That's all right. We'll be in touch with you later.'

By mid-November, I was worried. Now, there was nothing vague about the way I was feeling. I was getting intense pains across my midriff and while they lasted, they were agonising. Friends said: 'There's a tummy bug going the rounds.' I hoped that was all it was.

On the evening of Thursday, 16th November, Manchester City Council gave a Civic Reception for me, which is an honour rarely bestowed. As well as my personal guests, who included members of my family and two of my childhood friends, the Lord Mayor had invited city councillors, members of my Central Committee and representatives of the town hall staff, the Press and members of the Regional and Area Health Committees. It was a foul night as we headed in the direction of Manchester. On the motorway, torrential rain, strong winds, spray from other vehicles and poor visibility made driving conditions appalling. When we arrived at Manchester Town Hall. I was doubled up with pain and trying desperately to disguise the fact. Before the reception began, the Lord Mayor, Councillor Trevor Thomas, offered Geoff and me a drink. I asked for a neat whisky and surreptitiously took two pain killers with it. It would either 'fettle' me or flatten me! Fortunately, it worked. Within a quarter of an hour, the pain began to ease off and I could enjoy the very pleasant evening which had been arranged for me. The catering staff had put on a superb buffet. Among all the delicious, attractively presented food, was a gâteau, decorated with the words 'One in a Million'. I was very touched by the delectable efforts the girls had made for me, even though I wasn't up to eating much. It was yet another example of the many kindnesses shown to me and typical of the generosity of spirit behind the Appeal.

The following day, the pain was back again. This was no

'tummy bug'. I'd had more than a week of it and if that was all it was, it should have gone by now. It must be something more serious. But *what*? Was cancer on the rampage again? *What we are trying to do is to buy you some extra time . . .* January 1977 . . . I'd had twenty-two months. Maybe I couldn't expect much more. Oh, God, was my 'bonus' coming to an end?

I sat by the fire, in pain and in a state of depression, wondering what to do and reflecting on the events of the last two years. What was I in for? More surgery? More radiotherapy?

Oh, come on, girl! Pull yourself together! You keep telling people to seek help in time – take your own advice!

I rang my consultant at the Christie. Kindly as ever, his calm, matter-of-fact voice steadied my nerves as I answered his questions.

'It could very well be an ulcer. It's not uncommon. This sometimes happens with the drug you are on, especially when you've been taking it for some time. Come in and see me in the morning. Don't have any breakfast. I may decide to send you for barium X-rays.'

When Geoff came home and I told him he said it wasn't before time and the only sensible thing to do.

'D'you want me to come with you? You know I will, if you need me.'

I knew that he was due in court, on the bench, the following morning.

'Love, what could you do except sit there in Outpatients? No, Pauline has said she'll come, in case I don't feel like driving. I'm not worrying now. Going to the Christie is like going to my second home.'

Pauline settled herself in a chair in the Outpatients Department and opened the novel she was reading. As I left her, I said: 'Keep your fingers crossed for me.'

'I will. Good luck.'

An hour or so later, I rejoined her.

'What is it?' she asked.

I looked at the ceiling and tut-tutted.

'Duodenal ulcer – it's no wonder I've been creased with pain, is it?'

'That's the top executive's complaint. You're in fashion.'

'Fashion be blowed! They're welcome to them!'

As we were driving home along the motorway, I chuckled.

'What now?' asked Pauline.

'I don't know . . . life's ridiculous at times. In ordinary circumstances, one would be quite upset to find one had a duodenal ulcer. Here am I – thankful that's ALL it is. You've got to admit, it does have it's funny side. How about "Ulcer of the Year–MBE?" ' It was an idiotic thing to say, but relief can be as intoxicating as strong wine. The relief meant yet more pills, more medicine (never mind if I rattle, I'm still here).

Late November and an invitation to appear on 'Pebble Mill at One'. Pebble Mill is the BBC's Midlands Television Studio in Birmingham. Pam Creed, a member of the pro-gramme's production staff, asked that I be at the studio for 11 a.m. in preparation for the lunchtime magazine programme, on Thursday, 30th November. Pauline and I travelled down on Wednesday evening and stayed at an hotel.

'How many times is this that you've appeared on TV?'

I thought it was either ten or eleven. Counting repeats and excerpts, it was probably about twenty. The difficulty is that the subject is always the same. One has to find new things to say, find anecdotes and illustrations one hasn't used on pre-vious programmes. But then, that's journalism. TV is just another branch of it. It would be a long time before I would run out of things to tell about the remarkable things people had done. If writing them all would fill volumes as large as the *Encylopaedia Britannica*, telling them all would use up hours of television time.

I remember visiting a junior school in Manchester and after

talking to the children, I invited them to ask me questions. One little boy put up his hand and asked: 'What's it like, being on television?'

I'd smiled at him and replied: 'Like going to the dentist – nice when it's over!'

It's true. Not because I'm nervous. Funnily enough, television appearances don't throw me into a state of nerves. Every person watching is just one individual, and that's the person I'm talking to; and I'm so busy concentrating on remembering the sequences of the interviews, as they have previously been decided upon by whoever is interviewing me, that it is only afterwards that I am left wondering what sort of a job I have made of them. When they have been pre-recorded, and I see myself, I become hypercritical, thinking, I should have said this, or that; or, some point would have been more effective if put in a different way. However, once a programme is 'in the can', there's nothing one can do about it. With radio recordings, one can always erase the tape and start again. If the programme is 'live' then it's a 'one-off' and that's it.

It was St Andrew's Day and at Pebble Mill the band of the Black Watch Regiment was in the studio and opened the programme with a rousing Scottish march. Also on the programme was Ron Goodwin, composer of 'Those Magnificent Men in Their Flying Machines' and '633 Squadron' and many other well-known film scores. He and his wife Heather are super people. Not only did they hand me a donation for the Fund, Ron also said that if I thought he could help in any way, I'd to let him know. He also gave me one of his albums. It had '633 Squadron' on it and when I told him that Geoff had flown in Mosquitos during the war, he said, 'In that case, I'm not giving it to you. I'm giving it to your husband,' and autographed it for Geoff. That evening, my better half played it at full volume on our record player! Bob Langley interviewed me about the Fund and finally, the band of the Black Watch played Ron Goodwin's 'Aces High' with the composer conducting. When the programme was over, there were the usual eats and drinks. The sound engineers, the cameramen and the production staff had all spontaneously had separate whip rounds and they gave me their collections as their personal donations to the Fund. Pam Creed shook her head in disbelief. 'In all the time I've worked here, I've never known that happen before.'

Pauline and I were back in Garstang by tea time. At home, I unpacked my case and then repacked it, for the following morning Geoff and I were flying to the Isle of Man.

Attending two events in the Liverpool area, one Saturday in September, we had met Mr Bill Cain at the Orrell Park Social Club. Mr Cain is chairman of the Manx Variety Club and he'd said, 'Fix a date and come to the Island. We'll give you a super time and we'll put on a charity night for the Fund.' During our visit, I heard the Isle of Man described in various terms: 'Sixty-two thousand alcoholics clinging to a rock in the middle of the Irish Sea', which is somebody's idea of a joke about their licensing laws, more lenient than those of the mainland; and 'An Island of Myth and Magic', which is the one I prefer, for there was certainly a magical quality about the warmth of the welcome Geoff and I received.

We were flown from Blackpool to Ronaldsway by courtesy of British Island Airways. As we stepped on to the tarmac, Bill Cain and his wife Margaret were there to meet us, together with airport officials and Mr Jack Nivison, a member of the Legislative Council which is the Isle of Man Parliament – unique in that it is the oldest parliament in the world and in 1979 it celebrates its Millenium, a thousand years of continuous democratic government. The day began with coffee in the airport lounge and from then on, it was kindness all the way. At lunch at the Eagle Hotel, Port Erin, we met the President of the Manx Variety Club and his wife, Sir John and Lady Bolton, and also our host and hostess, Richard and

Joan Plant. We should have stayed the night at the Eagle, but events decreed otherwise.

A tour of the southern part of the Island preceded dinner, after which, Richard and Joan drove us to the Abbots Inn Club, Rushen Abbey, where a cabaret night in aid of the Fund was to be held. There were some very talented local artistes on the bill and British Midland Airways had flown in Pat Moriarty as top of the bill. Bill Cain and other members of the committee worked extremely hard. Bill compèred the show and auctioned several items, including a guitar which fetched £800.

I met and talked with Soroptimists of the Douglas Club and it was lovely to meet them again. But as the evening progressed, I began to feel unwell. Fighting down biliousness, I stuck it as long as I could, but eventually had to retire. Whether it was the ulcer, the past two days of travelling or just a straightforward tummy bug, I don't know, but I felt wretched. I hadn't been able to face the delicious supper and all I'd had to drink was tomato juice. I felt terrible, both physically and mentally, for I'd let everyone down when they'd been so kind and gone to such lengths to make us welcome. Geoff had to deputise for me by offering the words of thanks for the wonderful hospitality we had received and for the magnificent contributions to the Fund – totalling more than £2,250, from the Manx Variety Club and from the Soroptimists.

It was as much as I could do to pull myself together sufficiently to board the plane for Blackpool the next morning. By Saturday midday I was back in my own bed, hoping I would be well enough to keep a very special date on Monday afternoon – with Her Royal Highness Princess Alexandra.

If members of the Press were asked to vote for their favourite member of the Royal Family the Princess Alexandra would win the poll without question. Journalists and photographers are well aware that they are sometimes regarded as nuisances and many a self-important official, escorting some Royal person, has tried, contemptuously, to brush them aside. This Princess realises that they have a job of work to do. She goes out of her way to be accommodating, to make a photographer's work as easy as possible. She intuitively seems to understand that they have deadlines to meet and editors breathing down their necks.

Princess Alexandra is Chancellor of the University of Lancaster, and Monday, 4th December was degree day. Mr Ted Hindle, General Manager and Director of the *Lancaster Guardian* had written to ask Her Royal Highness if she would find it possible to present the Citizen of the Year Award.

This, the Princess had kindly agreed to do and it was arranged that she would arrive at Lancaster Town Hall at 4.40 p.m. following her visit to the University. Among those invited to the ceremony in the Mayor's Parlour were the representatives of many Lancaster organisations, totalling some sixty people. That day, the National Union of Journalists had called for strike action in support of a pay claim by all of their members working for provincial newspapers, of which the *Lancaster Guardian* is one. (It hardly affected me, for I'd little time to work at my own profession, strike or no strike.) It says much for the popularity of the Princess that every photographer was there and pickets kept away.

When the Princess arrived, Mr Scott and his wife Christine and my husband and I were introduced. Escorted by Mr Hindle, the Princess circulated among the guests, talking to each of them including my mother and my son. Mr Hindle then gave a short speech about the Citizen of the Year Award and asked the Princess to present me with the commemorative plaque, plus a ciné camera, projector and screen, which was the *Lancaster Guardian*'s gift to me. I then replied, quoting some examples of the support the Appeal had received from the people of the Lancaster area and thanking the Press,

Radio and Television for the invaluable assistance they had given to me. Finally, I thanked Mr Hindle for the superb present; the readers for nominating me Citizen of the Year and Her Royal Highness for making it such a memorable occasion for me.

With the formalities over, refreshments were served and guests began to talk and to circulate. Princess Alexandra said to me, 'Come on, let's sit down and have a chat.' She is so natural, so friendly, that one has to remind oneself to call her 'Ma'am' and it crossed my mind that in other circumstances, she is a woman I would be proud to have for my friend. However, Alexandra of Kent is a Royal Princess and I am – what I am. At one stage, seeing my mother standing alone, she'd told my son to 'go and look after your grandmother'. Later, as we talked, the Princess suggested that my mother join us. Her Royal Highness remarked that it was nice to see us together and said that she had been very close to her own mother, the late Princess Marina. I told her of the supportive role my family had played and how I could not have undertaken the work I was doing, had we not all worked together as a team.

The Princess was accompanied by her Lady in Waiting, Lady Mary Fitzalan Howard. Howard being my mother's name, she was delighted to tell Lady Mary that many years ago, she had read a book called *This Our Nobility* in which the name Howard was reputed to be the second oldest name in England. She could not remember which name was claimed to be the oldest.

When the occasion was over and the Princess had gone and as we were driving home, my mother said she would remember the day as long as she lived.

Like mother, like daughter, for indeed, so will I.

It had been a day to treasure.

12

The Young Travellers

'Children – A promise for the Future and a Blessing for today,' sings John Denver.

Throughout the Appeal, the children have been my delight. I have loved receiving their letters, more often than not written on Paddington Bear or Snoopy paper. I've been the receiver of confidences as well as donations. I've been made an honorary member of many a Secret Spy Club, on the strict understanding that I do not reveal to a living soul the pass-word, the code or chant. They have sent me painstakingly perfected paintings or drawings, poems or pressed flowers.

Spontaneously, groups of children – usually school friends – have got together to do something to help the Appeal and as a result, there has been many a back garden toy sale, or comic sale or jumble sale. Concerts have been held in garages, with Daddy's car exiled to the street to make room for the audiences, usually Mums and Dads, Aunties and Grannies.

Sally, aged ten, and her brother Simon, aged five-and-a-half, asked their Mummy if they could have a pancake party last Shrove Tuesday. Mummy agreed with the proviso that Sally and Simon did the washing up. They invited thirty of their little friends and Sally wrote to tell me: 'Mummy made

900 pancakes'! I did a double take when I read that. According to my arithmetic, that makes it about thirty pancakes per child. Either there were some very full children in Clitheroe or Sally had added a nought too many! I am sure their Mummy must have been worn out at the end of it all, for it is something of a marathon to make ninety pancakes, never mind 900.

But there have been times of sadness. I remember the letter I received telling me of the ten-year-old boy who had chopped and sold 5p bundles of firewood – because his Mummy had cancer . . . and to receive a letter from an eight- or nine-year-old, written in unformed handwriting and maybe with a few spelling mistakes, which says: 'My grannie has died of cancer and I want to help other grannies . . .' and which encloses the child's pocket-money, leaves you with an outsize lump in your throat.

I remember at a primary school in Bolton being presented with a cheque by an eight-year-old boy. Standing next to him was his little brother of six who had just been diagnosed as having leukemia. Situations like this take all one's self-control.

About the most harrowing experience involving a child, happened at Chorley, in the summer of 1978. That particular day was one of my 'off' days. To start with, it was an effort to fulfil that engagement and I'd have given anything to have stayed at home and gone to bed. However, I got there, and during the course of the afternoon, I was presented with some flowers by a little tiny girl in a dainty smocked dress who was also wearing a spotless white frilly mob cap. I had my suspicions when I saw that mob cap, for the day wasn't particularly sunny. Then I was told that this little two-year-old mite was a cancer patient. She was suffering from cancer of the kidney and the treatment, as is often the case, had caused her to lose her hair

How I managed to accept those flowers and pose for pictures for the local papers, I just do not know, for inside of me my heart was breaking. However, in January 1979 her Mummy reported that little Claire was doing fine. And yet, in a way, such experiences have kept me going. They have renewed the fury and given me the extra stamina I have needed to continue the pace. For little ones like these, I'd move heaven and earth to give them the hope of a better future, a better chance in life. If that scanner helps at least some of these little ones, all that I or anyone else has done to help get it installed, has been time well spent. For little children, I will fight every inch of the way. I should think there is hardly a school in the north-west which hasn't made some contribution. It would be impossible to mention them all. Suffice to say that in total, their offerings must have added a six-figure sum to the Fund. Equally as important, I have found that children and young people are now using the word 'cancer' freely and in a matter-of-fact way. The younger generation are bringing the word out from under the carpet. If, as a result, they gain a better understanding of it and in the process, lose some of the fear which surrounds the word, then the chances are that as they grow up, their more enlightened attitude will mean that they will not hesitate to seek medical advice, should they feel it is necessary. For children don't raise money without wanting to know what it is for and why it is needed. If schools have used the fund-raising to throw in some cancer education at the same time it can do nothing but good.

Following national publicity, donations have come from schools in many parts of Britain – from, for example, Crammond School, Edinburgh; Holemead School, Biggleswade; Carshalton High School; Radyr Comprehensive, Cardiff; Twickenham Girls' School; and again, it would be impossible to name them all. I have been extremely impressed by the enterprise these young people have shown, for their fund-raising ideas have been far from stereotyped. When I was a girl at Tootal Road School, Salford, I was in Nightingale

House. My old school has now been superseded by Hope High School and you can imagine my delight when the children of Nightingale House sent donations to the fund and what a sentimental journey it was for me when I visited the school.

One school has paid me just about the nicest compliment I have ever received. They don't have 'houses' at St Michael's C of E High School, Chorley. Instead, they have 'tutorials' which are named after people. Headmaster Mr R. Moore wrote to tell me that those tutorials already in existence are named after people such as Gladys Aylward, Doctor Barnardo, Kathleen Ferrier and Helen Keller's teacher, Anne Sullivan. The trouble is, said Mr Moore, 'most of the people one might think of are no longer living. Hence, when we have the opportunity to help the children to identify in a more personal way with the Patron of their Group, we try to arrange a meeting.' St Michael's now has a Pat Seed Tutorial. I am to meet them next month and I hope this Patron lives long enough to get to know them and be of some use to them.

We hear so much about vandalism and delinquency. In my opinion, they stem from lack of adult interest and lack of love. But my overall impression of the younger generation as I have met and talked with them in the course of this Appeal, is that we have some fine young boys and girls on the way up, who will be the caring, responsible citizens of the next few decades. In a world that is fraught with troubles and stresses of one kind and another, these young people have made me feel that we can view the future of Britain with optimism and hope. I thank them for all that they have done to help me and for the concern they have so significantly demonstrated. I wish them well, for they are indeed, our promise for the future and our blessing for today.

13

Team Work

Although the Appeal is geared to equip a north-west hospital with a piece of technology, support for it has come from many places in Britain and beyond. As well as individual people, whole communities have taken it to their hearts: communities in their places of work; communities in their places of residence; communities in schools.

Let's take a look at some of these combined efforts, to find how some of them have interpreted the word 'community' and how it has affected their lives. 'Community' has reared its benign head in many firms, be it an office swear box, a social occasion or a full-scale event. The staffs of chain stores, such as Marks & Spencer, British Home Stores, Woolworths, C & A, Lewis's have all played their part and made very substantial contributions. If Lewis's in Blackpool gave us counter space to sell badges, Lewis's in Manchester did things on a grand scale. In the spring of 1978 they staged a North-West Genius Exhibition on the store's fifth floor and devoted a whole window on Market Street to the Christie Hospital and the Scanner. It was a first-rate exhibition, and expertly staged. Many notable north-west firms displayed examples of their technology and expertise and the walls were lined with pictures and biographical notes on eminent north-west people, past and present. I was glad to see that my journalistic hero, Charles Prestwich Scott, was included. Many thousands of the 'community' came to see the exhibition and it raised several thousands of pounds for the Fund. As I stood on the platform with the Lord Mayor of Manchester on the day the exhibition was opened, I couldn't help but reflect that this was the very spot to which my mother had brought me at the age of three, to see Father Christmas and the fairy grotto. A lot of water has gone under the River Irwell bridge since then. Now, I was standing there in a quite different role and had motivated an exhibition which demonstrated to the community at large, just how much the people of the north-west had achieved of which they could be justifiably proud.

The firm of Proctor and Gamble have factories all over the world. They have one in Trafford Park, Manchester. Each year, the firm gives a cash prize as a Safety Award to that one of their factories where the employees have had the least time off work due to accidents. In 1978, the Trafford Park factory won it and the staff unanimously decided to forgo their hand-out and donate the money to the Appeal. They presented me with a cheque for £2,000 and this was in addition to a cheque for about £1,500 from their Sports and Social Club.

Following a broadcast on British Forces Network support came in from Germany, Holland, Acritiri and all places where our services are stationed. For example, more than one British Forces school in Germany has sent a four-figure cheque – the result of the servicemen's children doing sponsored walks.

Two 'community' events took place in the Lancaster area and one of them won international recognition. The first was organised in Caton, a small village to the east of Lancaster. Instead of holding a series of individual events spread over a long period, the people of Caton chose to hold one week of concerted effort. During that week, every single organisation in the village held some function, with even the Toddlers'

Club holding a sponsored jelly eating contest. Can you imagine that? I wish I'd been there to see it. However, I did go to meet some of those kindly people one night in their village hall, when they presented me with their cheque, which was for more than £2,000. In addition, they gave me a very pleasant and friendly evening.

In January of last year I was invited to speak to the members of the Rotary Club of Lunesdale. The members had it in mind to organise something in support of the Fund, but first they wanted the fullest information about the scanner, the Fund and me. I gave them as much detail as I could and answered any questions they asked. The Rotarians decided they would arrange a mammoth Sponsored Swim, involving as many local schools as possible. As a result of this engagement, I was invited to Casterton School at Kirkby Lonsdale. In the school hall I spoke to the assembled pupils, and headmaster Mr Tom Penny left it to the girls themselves to decide how they would help me. Later in the year, they held their own sponsored swim in the school pool as part of Lunesdale Rotary's effort. Just before the school broke up for its summer holidays, I again visited Casterton. The result of their swim and the generosity of their sponsors enabled them to give me a cheque for more than £3,000. I was also invited to open their new domestic science block which I did with pleasure. In the pool at Hornby, school children from all over the district swam. It involved gargantuan organisation and it took a considerable time for sponsor money of this magnitude to be collected. However, on 10th November, just ten months after I had first met the members, the Rotary Club of Lunesdale invited Geoff and me to be their guests at dinner at Melling Hall. After an excellent meal, they presented their cheque – £7,121. Together with the contribution from Casterton, it made a grand total of more than £10,000. It brought the club international recognition with a special commendation from Rotary International Headquarters in America.

BBC Radio Blackburn have a monthly programme 'People in Their Places'. In March 1978, Judith Roberts visited the village of Freckleton to find out what effect supporting the Appeal had on the community. Judith first interviewed Mrs Norma Fenton, who said that she had attended a meeting of the Weightwatchers Organisation in Blackpool when I was presented with a cheque for £500. She had come home and put on her thinking cap. She held a clothes party in the village's new Memorial Hall which raised £100. Following this, she realised that if every organisation in the village would each do something, they could really go places. A meeting was held, various ideas were put forward, most of which were put into practice. Within ten weeks, Freckleton had raised £4,000, the largest event being a 'Pat Seed Weekend' which included a Grand Military and Services Display and a Spring Fair in which the entire village took part.

Talking to the chairman of the parish council, Mr Harry Robinson, Judith said that she understood that until then, there hadn't been much community spirit in Freckleton. Mr Robinson said that they had some problems in the past. The Queen's Silver Jubilee celebrations had helped to some extent, but the Appeal had meant that people had worked together for a common cause. It had meant that many had met and shaken hands with people they had not previously known, and now a wider net could be cast to draw people into village community life.

Judith then talked with Mr Alan Jepson, the Methodist Youth Leader, whose wife Glynis had suffered an unfortunate experience because the Christie *didn't* have a scanner. In order to define the extent of cancer of her lymphatic system, Glynis had to lie on her back for five hours as dyes and oily liquids were injected, which would show up on ordinary X-rays. It was a far from pleasant experience.

'I would like to think that future patients won't have to

undergo this additional stress at a time which is very worrying for them. With the scanner, it would have been a comparatively quick and painless procedure.' Mr Jepson then went on to say that not only his own youth club, but every young persons' organisation in the village had become involved with an enthusiasm he had never known before. There had been far more enjoyment and effort than for anything else in all his experience of Freckleton. Roy Kiddle was born and bred in Freckleton and over the years he's seen the village grow as new housing estates were built. Judith asked him if he thought the Appeal would put its mark on the village and he replied: 'Yes, I definitely do. Now that something has brought people together, I think the people of Freckleton will want it to stay that way.' Thus spoke four people who are members of the Freckleton branch of the Appeal Fund.

In Burnage, on the outskirts of Manchester, Mr Leslie Jones is the headmaster of Acacias County Primary School. One of his pupils was a child of eleven years, academically clever, with the promise of a brilliant future ahead of her. Jane Butler was also a good all rounder at games and was a leading light of the school's netball team. When this popular little girl died of cancer, it shocked the whole school and it motivated pupils, parents and people in the surrounding community to raise money for the scanner in memory of Jane. For the saddest of reasons, nearly £10,000 has been added to the Fund.

In the village of Endmoor near Kendal, Cumbria, the community got together to help the Appeal and formed a branch of the Fund. The reason? Again, a sad one. Seven-year-old Ian Irvine was found to have a brain tumour and at his parents' wish, a committee was formed. Little Ian died, but the people of Endmoor have done what they can so that others like him may have the hope of a future. Few realise that between birth and fourteen years of age, cancer is responsible for more deaths than anything other than accidents. Some people are not even aware that children *can* have cancer.

Jessie Andrew is treasurer of a small committee formed in the little community of Whaley Bridge, near Macclesfield. In a recent letter, Jessie told me that when they first decided to help the Appeal, they called a meeting at the Rectory and then wrote to every organisation in the village – Roman Catholic and Methodist churches, Church of England people, guides, scouts, WI and Townswomen's Guild, Red Cross, Liberal, Labour and Conservative Clubs, etc. – and asked if they would each send a representative to a meeting to decide what could be done. When the various organisations met together, they decided they would hold a Spring Fair, with each of them manning a stall. It was a lovely spring day and Whaley Bridge had never seen anything like it before.

'People were almost fighting to get into the hall, it was so packed. All the different organisations worked together and really enjoyed it. It was almost unheard of, here, to have all the denominations working together for a common cause and we all thoroughly enjoyed ourselves.'

Following the Spring Fair, the villagers held four very successful 'food container' parties, three jumble sales and other events which amounted to a grand total of over two and a half thousand pounds.

'Apart from raising money,' says Jessie, 'It was so good to get local people together in this way, for there is little social activity in Whaley Bridge. There had never ever been anything like this before to capture the interest of the entire community. Everyone has worked so well together and given whatever they have to give.'

Like Freckleton, the east Lancashire village of Barrowford has expanded over the years. Some eight years ago, a new estate was built of some thirty to forty properties. When they were completed they were occupied by all age groups, but mostly by young married couples, some of whom had children. The older residents were either retired or on the point of retiring. The inhabitants lived their separate lives, and for the first seven years had little more than a nodding acquaintance with each other. Life in Shap Close, Barrowford, was insular and at times, lonely.

About a year ago, all that changed. It began to change when a Mrs Roma Nutter (no connection with the comedy act) decided she'd have a coffee evening for the Appeal Fund. She invited her neighbours and it proved so enjoyable that it inspired another Shap Close housewife, Mrs Marjorie Massey, to hold a Christmas Evening. Marjorie made Christmas cake and mince pies; there was a small present on the Christmas tree for everyone and she played Christmas music and carols on her record player. Added to all this, there was a bring-and-buy stall and by the time this pleasant evening ended, the ladies were beginning to know each other better. They began to think what each of them could do, both to help the Appeal and further the friendships which were being formed. The result, during 1978 a lot of events were organised, including a jewellery party, a sponsored slim, a cheese and wine party, a Lancashire Lass evening, Groceries Galore.

By high summer I was told that Shap Close was a different place. It had become a friendly community and the ladies invited me to open their Bargain Bonanza in the hall of the parish church of St Thomas. When Geoff and I arrived, the hall was packed and on a variety of stalls there were a wide selection of items for sale. After the opening formalities, they presented me with flowers and a silver plated tray which they'd had inscribed with the words 'Pat Seed, One in a Million'. One of the girls said to me: 'You don't know what you've done for us. Before we started working for the Appeal, none of us knew each other. Now, we're all good friends.'

I replied, 'I haven't done anything for you. You've done it for yourselves. All you needed was a good reason to break through that typically British reserve. Once you'd lost that, you found that you had as much to offer to each other as you had to offer to the Fund.'

By the end of November, just a year after that first coffee evening, the ladies of Shap Close sent me their cheque for all their efforts. It came to £1,544. In raising this money, they had formed friendships which are continuing. The younger adults keep a watchful eye on the older generation, helping where they can. They baby-sit for each other's children. Life is richer and fuller and all say they have reaped a lasting benefit of a kind which cannot be bought with money.

Mrs Evans, who chaired the organisation behind the Bargain Bonanza, gave a party for them all, both as a 'thank you' and as a celebration. It included competitions for paper masks and a home-made Christmas decoration. These were judged by Linda Hardman, a journalist with the *Nelson Leader and Colne Times* newspaper.

One of the ladies told me: 'Being rather shy, for seven years I didn't know anyone. Now, I can knock on anyone's door and know that I will get a welcome.'

That's what 'community' is all about and it's been one of the finest spin-offs of the Appeal.

14

The Route Mappers

The work of the Central Committee of the Appeal Fund has been of vital importance and I am deeply indebted to the men who have given their time to it, for theirs have been the decisions, theirs the responsibility. When the committee first met on 10th October 1977, it was something of a 'getting to know you' exercise. Although many had met previously in connection with other interests, this was the first occasion when we had met as a team.

As I have mentioned elsewhere, election of the committee's officers took place; two consultants and two lay members were nominated as Trustees of the Fund and there was considerable discussion as to the role of the committee. For the benefit of members, the consultants readily agreed to produce information about Computerised Axial Tomography and in particular, about the system installed at the University Medical School, so that all members were fully briefed. We also decided that a 'statement of intent' should be sought from the Regional Health Authority and from the Manchester Area Health Authority. We needed to know exactly where we stood with them; whether the Appeal and its objectives had their blessing and to try to ascertain what measure of co-operation could be expected. At that first meeting, the Fund total was then £110,000.

I think that when the Appeal was launched, those in authority had viewed me either as some crank who was trying to start a minor revolution, or as an enthusiastic patient who was full of good intentions, but who had about as much chance of getting a CAT scanner for the Christie as primeval man had of going to the moon. They were not alone in this thinking.

With the Fund in six figures in less than seven months, the powers that be were beginning to sit up and take notice. They had to. The Appeal was not only gaining financially day by day, it was gaining in popularity as men and women from all walks of life chose to identify with it. Someone, somewhere, was going to have to decide just what the 'official' attitude should be.

Now, it wasn't just some enthusiastic patient wanting to know the answers, it was a group of highly respected men of stature, astuteness and experience asking the questions and they were led by the Lord Lieutenant of Greater Manchester.

At this inaugural meeting, the Central Committee discussed the campaign programme; the need to co-opt more members on to the committee and the desirability of Patrons for the Appeal. As it happened, the latter question was soon resolved and without too much difficulty, for a few days later I met Ken Dodd, and Sir William talked with Sir Matt Busby. Both readily agreed to be Patrons of the Fund. That first meeting lasted two hours and during that time, a lot of ground was covered. I came away considerably heartened by what had been achieved and impressed by the purposeful, constructive way in which discussions had proceeded. It was a load off my mind. I was no longer alone. I had some of the best brains available to guide the project around or over the innumerable obstacles which would undoubtedly present themselves. The responsibility no longer rested entirely on my shoulders; these were men who could speak with authority and, should it be necessary, argue from strength.

The committee met for the second time on 3rd November and the Fund total had then reached £150,000. It was at this meeting we proposed to arrange a meeting of the branch committees of the Fund in late January of 1978. (Again, I cannot overstress the importance of the branch meeting, for it gave the branch representatives an opportunity to meet members of the Central Committee – many of whom had just been 'names' to them; equally, it gave members of the Central Committee a chance to meet the people 'in the field' and to observe for themselves the degree of dedication and sense of purpose that existed.) At this second meeting, Mr Geoffrey Ball, manager of Garstang Nat-West, was asked to assume the role of financial adviser as well as that of Fund Treasurer. This he has done, and it is worthy of note that he has been able to call upon the expertise of the National Westminster Bank, not only at Regional level, but also that of London headquarters staff. Again, the best brains in banking were at the disposal of the Fund. At this meeting, I reported that I had been approached by a professional fund raiser. Since the fund raiser would retain forty per cent of any monies he raised, the idea was strongly rejected and I was fully in agreement with the decision.

The Central Committee also decided that at this stage discussions with the Manchester Area Health Authority and the Regional Health Authority should be informal and confidential. What we were seeking was co-operation and goodwill. Far more can be achieved by such methods than by publicity ridden confrontations and again, I was glad about this (with the proviso that there would be no dragging of feet), for the whole Appeal was founded on goodwill and I wanted to keep it that way.

The question of a building in which the scanner could be housed was discussed. The Christie is like Topsy – it just growed! What originated as a twenty-bed home for cancer incurables was now the largest cancer treatment centre in Europe, with the Patterson laboratories and a new block of four double wards, plus a reception area and extra theatres taking up much of any spare space which might at one time have been available. It would be advantageous and make for easier and more efficient treatment if the new facility could be positioned as near as possible to those already in existence. It was arranged that the three consultants on the committee, plus Mr Roy Fisher, a consultant architect, should do a preliminary survey to decide the best and most convenient site for the new department.

Their meeting took place within the next week and the old entrance hall, which was now virtually the 'back door' of the hospital plus the stretch of tarmac in front of it, at present being used as a car park, was found to be the best site. It was adjacent to the 'business end' of the hospital and near to X-ray diagnostics, radium treatment theatres and the radiotherapy department. The old foyer would become the reception area of the new department with the department itself extending on to the former car park. To this scheme the firm of consultant architects who usually undertake building projects at the Christie readily agreed.

I do not intend to detail every minutiae of every meeting of the Central Committee. Suffice to say that a great deal of hard work – investigation, consultation and negotiation – took place over the months. Problems arose. They were discussed. Decisions were made and the problems dealt with. In all my experience of committees, I have never known any that measured up to the Central Committee of the Fund; they were purposeful, constructive, progressive and with no 'waffling' whatsoever. Busy people don't have the time to waffle.

By April of 1978 we knew that the Area and the Regional Health Authorities had agreed to accept the Appeal Fund's gift of a CAT scanner for the Christie. There were, however, certain conditions. It had been made clear that the Fund not only had to meet the capital installation consequences, it would have to finance the whole scheme for a ten-year period – *in its entirety*. This meant that in addition to maintaining the scanner and the building, the Fund must find the money to meet staffing costs – wages and salaries – of all the personnel employed in the new department.

At the end of April, the Fund reached the original target figure of three quarters of a million pounds. Another milestone along the 'Trail', but the edge was taken off any celebrations because by now we knew that this wasn't going to be enough. Estimates which were eighteen to twenty months old were now obsolete. The whole scheme had been hit by inflation; technology was advancing rapidly. Dr Hounsfield's invention, marketed by EMI, now had competition. Other firms were producing CAT scanners and EMI were making improvements on earlier models.

It is just like motor cars, washing machines, television sets – someone invents them and puts a prototype on the market. The next thing you know, a dozen or more firms are producing their version of the same product. We had reached the 'second generation' of scanners. They were more sophisticated; they did the job faster and with better imagery. They were also far more expensive. When you are thinking of spending this sort of money – a vast sum, donated by ordinary people in good faith, you need to be pretty damned certain that what you buy is the best possible purchase at that time. It is a tremendous responsibility and not one to take lightly. The technical members of the committee would need to inspect all the scanners on the market if they were to make a thorough investigation and assessment. So, for a time, the question of 'which scanner' was an open-ended question. Until that question was resolved, and we knew how much the scanner to be chosen would cost and what sort of a package deal it would involve, we could not say how much money we needed. There were other factors too; how much had inflation increased the cost of the building? The building was as much a piece of technology as the scanner itself and architects were busy having plans drawn. These could not be finally approved or quantity surveyed and costed until we knew which scanner, for the design might have to be amended according to the specifications of the scanner chosen.

It made it very difficult, not only from the point of view of the Central Committee but from the point of view of those of us who met the members of the public and members of clubs and organisations who were working so hard to raise money. The inevitable question was, 'How much do you need?' and unfortunately, at this point, there was no simple answer. It would have been easy for us if there had been a figure to quote, instead of having to repeat, times without number, just what the position was and why we couldn't give a figure. Any figure quoted could only be inspired guesswork at the best.

The other thundering big question mark – and I have to admit that it hangs over me like the sword of Damocles – is how much money will be needed to meet wages and salaries for the next ten years? It would take a clairvoyant to even hazard a guess at that one and it is why we cannot, however much we might wish to, put a ceiling figure on this Fund. I sometimes reflect, if I had known when I started all this, just what an astronomical sum of money would be needed – would I have had the temerity to even begin? I am a natural optimist, but I wonder if even I could have been *that* optimistic. I admit that there have been times when I have found this constant need for yet more money daunting and depressing. Then some kind person has written or telephoned and what they have told me has given me new heart to persevere.

Among all these unanswered questions, decisions still to be made, factors unresolved, there was one bright note. The Regional Health Authority decreed that we could make a start even though we had not yet enough money to meet the costs of the entire project. We could go ahead with the building; we could plan for the installation of the scanner while at the same time continue to raise money to meet the rest of our obligations. I know . . . I can almost hear you saying, 'That's big of them!'

I feel that it is only fair to say something about the North-West Regional Health Authority. If I and the Appeal are Red Riding Hood, the Authority is certainly not cast in the role of the Big Bad Wolf.

Central Government allows the Regional Health Authority a sum of money each year. It is never enough. The Region then has to allocate it among all the hospitals in the Region, according to the needs of each hospital and as a matter of priority. Needless to say, the annual budget does not meet every need and, quite naturally, every hospital hopes that its particular needs will be somewhere near the top of the priority list. When the RHA has to make cuts, or even close parts of some hospitals, they do so with regret, but such measures are a genuine attempt to make the best and most efficient use of resources available.

Even gifts can be an embarrassment. Let's take a hypothetical example. Say some charitable organisation, having raised a sum of money, wants to buy an ambulance for a particular hospital or home in their locality. All very creditable, you might say. And it *is* – but the Area Health Authority or the Regional Health Authority then has to find and pay the salary of a driver for that ambulance; someone to maintain it; somewhere to garage it, maybe. All of these things will cost money which the Authority hasn't got and for which it hasn't budgeted.

On a larger scale, this is exactly the problem the Appeal Fund faces. The DHSS bought the scanner at Manchester University Medical School, but it is funded out of the Regional budget. The annual allocation from Central Government is such that they just haven't the resources to fund another. If I have any personal criticisms – and I stress that what I am about to say are purely personal opinions – they are not levelled at Regional Government, but at Central Government in Westminster. Nor, as a citizen of a democratic country, am I afraid to voice them. The people at Westminster are the people we, the population, have elected to represent us. If we do not agree with the way they handle things, we have the freedom to say so.

In my opinion and for far too long, the north-west has been the poor relation when it comes to handouts from Central Government via the National Health Service. I well remember that in October 1977 the Minister of Health during the Labour Party Conference in Brighton, was interviewed on TV and he stated that he intended to make more money available for Health Services in the north-west. True to his word, he has done so. In 1978/9 the region had a growth rate of four per cent in its annual revenue. In view of what needs to be done, it's about as much use as an extra teaspoonful of salt water in the Irish Sea. One has to be philosophical. Anything is better than nothing. The Minister admits that because the region has been so badly deprived of resources in the past, it is going to take quite some time before all the needs which have been identified in the region are met.

But when one reflects that millions of pounds have been injected into British industries, many of which, in spite of this extra money, still show an annual deficit, and that millions of pounds owed by overseas countries have been wiped off the slate – WHAT is four per cent? Viewed in this context, a direct grant of £100,000 to this Appeal Fund would be nothing more than peanuts.

If I were a politician – and thank heavens I'm not! – I think I would have been quick to appreciate how encouraging the people of the north-west would have viewed such a gift and been aware of the fact that it could also have been worth a few north-west votes at the next general election.

I am not a mathematician or a statistician. One doesn't need to be to take in the significance of the following figures. At the close of 1978 there were fifteen EMI whole body scanners installed in Britain. Ten are in the London area. Nine more are on order and two of those are for hospitals within the London Health Authority areas. Of the thirty-eight brain scanners EMI has installed in the UK, fifteen are within the London area.

Some of these machines have been bought outright by benefactors; others have been partially paid for by benefactors or by public subscription, supplemented by government money.

As far as the people of the north-west are concerned, there is nothing new in this. But, in our Lancashire dialect, we have a saying, 'If tha' does owt for nowt, do it for thissel.' In finding money for the Christie CAT scanner, they have done just this and it's been a first-rate do-it-yourself job. We have had assistance from people from other parts of Britain, from British Forces overseas and from wellwishers abroad, but the bulk of the money has come from the north-west as a direct result of that northern independence of spirit. I identify with it and I am proud of it. Proud? Yes, for although I would have liked to see some help forthcoming from the government as a token of recognition, I do not subscribe to the maxim that we be cushioned by the State from the cradle to the grave. By that, I do not mean that there should be no State welfare (as opposed to Welfare State). Nobody should be allowed to starve, nobody should be without shelter and everyone should have access to an efficient medical service. Like many other people, I view with abhorrence the misuse of DHSS facilities and social benefits. But if the State were to provide every last thing we need, it could be detrimental. It could sap initiative, leave us without the incentive or the will to get up and do things for ourselves. Therefore – and this is where I agree with the Minister of Health – voluntary organisations DO have a very important part to play. Especially in the present economic climate. State provision, with voluntary organisations to supplement the needs. There is room for both and somewhere along the line is a happy medium. Just where that line should be drawn is a matter for endless conjecture and debate.

However, I cannot hide my disappointment that Central Government have not recognised the sterling work that ordinary people have done in raising over one and a half million pounds for the Appeal Fund. It should be remembered that when that new department is operational at the Christie, it becomes the property of Government, via the Manchester Area Health Authority.

Having got that off my chest, let me return to the work of the Central Committee.

By the end of March 1978, the consultants had made several visits to Europe in the course of their normal work. They had taken the opportunity to inspect several scanner installations in Germany and Holland. There remained the installations on the other side of the Atlantic and reports coming from the United States about some of those sounded very promising indeed. Also, in EMI's Chicago factory, their latest technology was nearing completion. All members of the Central Committee were aware that we owed it to the people who were providing the money to make certain that the Christie got the very best CAT system available. The only way to make sure of that was for the consultants to go to the States on a fact-finding visit. Every manufacturer's brochure or marketing campaign extols the virtues of his product. That applies whether the product is a brand of soap powder or a jumbo jet 'plane. The only way our consultants could make a true evaluation was to go and see for themselves. The Central Committee affirmed that the cost should be met from Fund interest.

In June, Doctors Todd, Eddleston and Greene spent a week

in the United States, visiting hospitals and clinics, gleaning information and technical data at first hand. Although they found the visit interesting in the extreme, the pace was exhausting. On their return, they began their evaluation which involved several meetings at the Christie in addition to their normal professional duties. After many hours of discussion, they narrowed the field down to three installations.

Again, it's like buying a car or a washing machine – no one model has absolutely everything. You may like the bodywork on one car, the gear box on another; miles per gallon or power-assisted steering may be important to you. The customer will choose after considering what each manufacturer has to offer and which, as near as possible, meets his requirements. Of the final three firms in the running, there was very little to choose between them, but one factor tipped the scales in favour of EMI. Discussions were held with the representatives of the DHSS, the Manchester University, the Regional Physics Department and the Christie Radiotherapy staff. It was agreed that the specification of EMI's 7070 treatment planning unit was considerably ahead of its competition. The Christie were buying British – and now we *could* afford it.

Can you imagine my elation? I had hoped against hope that the British model would be chosen, but common sense decreed that the consultants must make a completely unbiased opinion. This they had done. The scientific research and most of the component parts of EMI's 7070 were produced in Britain, though some parts and the actual assembly took place in Chicago.

The Emiscanner 7070, together with its treatment planning system, would be the first of its kind to be installed in a British hospital. It meant that the new department at the Christie would be the finest purpose-built Computerised Axial Tomography Department in the world. *This* was the pay-off for all our hard work, all the coffee mornings, sponsored events, etc., which had made it possible.

So let's take a look at the Emiscanner 7070. What have the manufacturers to say about it?

The earlier 'Emi' whole body scanner takes 20 seconds to scan a 'slice'. The new 7070 picks up a million and a half readings, in just three seconds and presents the scan information in uncompromised picture quality, thus giving unparalleled diagnostic scope. This unprecedented scan speed and superlative imagery opens up new areas of CAT application. It allows maximum patient comfort and has finer, faster and simpler control. It is the most advanced CAT system yet devised. The key to EMI Medical's diagnostic breakthrough is revolutionary. It's called Mutating Sensor Geometry – an elegantly simple engineering solution to a problem as old as CAT technology. The Emiscanner 7070 overcomes the traditional incompatibility between high scan speed and high picture quality. It offers new horizons in diagnostic application and control. Angled scans which at one time could not have been contemplated for certain patients may now be simply undertaken by means of gantry tilt (plus ten degrees to minus thirty degrees) and patient table slew (plus or minus twenty degrees). The operator is free to select any one of five scan times and five scan fields from 120 mm to 500 mm.

I am not attempting to blind the reader with science. I couldn't. I'm not a scientist. But perhaps the above will give some indication of the value of this wonder of modern medical scientific research and engineering technology.

Meanwhile, the Christie had acquired a machine known as a Simulator. This had been paid for with the hospital's allocation of regional funds. Although it was already in use, it was decided that it could be used to greater effect if it were to be incorporated in the new department, when it was built.

In an endeavour to explain its purpose as simply as possible I again resort to a bit of graphic journalese. The system is rather like using a dress pattern on a piece of material. Only in this case, the 'pattern' is for the accurate positioning of treatment areas on the patient's body. And as with a dress pattern, it may be used again and again, for the simulator will reproduce the treatment plan instantly – thus saving much repetitive work. In consequence, there is a faster throughput of patients. It will mean that the new CAT department will handle twenty to twenty-five patients a day, instead of the expected ten per day.

Now that the make of scanner had been selected, plans for the building could be finalised. Looking to the future, and the ever-escalating construction costs, the Central Committee considered it would be prudent that the single-storey department be designed with sufficient strength to take an upper storey at some future date. It would add a relatively small sum to the present price, whereas in two, three or five years' time, it might very well cost what amounted to a small fortune.

Fixed price tenders were invited from six building firms and the project was costed and quantity surveyed. The tender of William Thorpe & Son Limited was accepted. Some of our engineering specifications were still subject to confirmation. Therefore, a margin against possible additional expenditure was thought advisable, and the Central Committee approved the sum of a quarter of a million pounds to cover all construction work.

The scanner itself would cost almost half a million pounds. However, just as one has to spend money on having a motor car serviced and purchase spare parts for it, an annual sum would have to be set aside to service the scanner. This, it was estimated, would take about £39,000 per annum. For ten years, it means a sum of £390,000 must be earmarked for the purpose. That takes care of £1,140,000. Frightening, isn't it? And that's before one has even begun to think about wages and salaries. Over ten years, those could average £65,000 per annum, making the arithmetic total £1,790,000. At that, it provides no leeway for unexpected contingencies. For who can predict, with any degree of certainty, what wages and salaries will be in ten years' time? Nobody. With imponderables such as this, any figures quoted can at best be no more than inspired guesswork. The only thing about which we are certain, is that this Fund has to stand the total cost.

Although by September, the decision on 'which scanner' had been made, it was not made public knowledge until 4th November 1978. On that date, we held a second meeting of representatives of the Branch Committees at the Christie, and the Central Committee – quite rightly – took the view that they should be acquainted with the facts before a press release made it public knowledge.

Some eighty people attended this meeting and there was a buoyancy, an aura of success about it. When we all stood on the site and the building plans were explained, everyone of us felt that we were on the brink of seeing the dream become a reality. *This* was what we had all worked for. Now, it was all about to happen, for the builders were taking over the site on 11th December. It was scheduled for completion by 31st August 1979. After a few weeks of testing the highly complicated apparatus, the Christie's CAT Department would go into action in the autumn and the future would look a whole lot brighter and more hopeful for many of the hospital's patients.

It was a great step forward in cutting that old ogre, Cancer, down to size, and those words of Professor Luxton, which I had quoted in my original *Gazette* articles, began to assume a prophetic quality.

15

In Sight of the Summit

Early in December 1978, I went to the Christie for my monthly medical check, packing into the day four other business appointments.

The ulcer was beginning to subside and the verdict was 'so far, so good'.

'You're still putting on weight,' remarked my consultant.

'Goodness knows why. I'm not terribly interested in food. It's not through over-eating.'

'No, the drug may be partially responsible.'

'How long do you think I will be taking it, always supposing things continue to go well?' Then I looked at his expression and said: 'Forget it – that's not a fair question, is it? I'll stick to my recipe – one day at a time.'

'It's the only way, Pat.'

A few minutes later, I was hurrying along the corridor to the old entrance hall of the Christie, which is to be the reception area of the new department. The previous day, the building firm had taken over the site. I met and talked with one of their directors and the site foreman. The site was now clear of all the cars which normally parked there (where did they put them?) and the ground already marked out.

Using my new ciné camera, I took some film for the record, for the porticoed entrance, with the flight of steps leading to the tarmac forecourt, would never look the same again. Now, it was all about to happen . . . Having lived, thought, breathed, ate and slept 'Scanner' all these eventful months, the project was about to become a reality. Here was I, standing in the pouring rain, on the very spot where the scanner would be . . . 'Pinch me, somebody, and I'll wake up!' The building was about to be started. Telling myself that to anyone passing along the corridor, I must look a fool, standing there, getting soaked, I came out of my reverie and went to the Hospital Secretary's office.

We discussed a foundation-stone laying ceremony. We thought a Monday in January would be suitable and, conferring by telephone with the architects, suggested either the 15th or 22nd. After some discussion we settled for the 22nd.

The following morning, I was telling Pauline about the various conversations I'd had at the Christie. She has often remarked that 'Someone' is watching over this Appeal.

'Whenever we've been stumped and don't know what to do for the best, somehow, the answer always seems to be handed to us on a plate. There have been far too many coincidences over the months to take them all for granted.'

I gazed at her over the rim of my coffee cup. There she was, sitting at my desk with her cup of coffee. On the desk was her typewriter and all the office paraphernalia and the day's letters.

'Coincidences? How about this one? I've just realised – on the day that stone is laid, it will be just two years to the very day since I tottered out of that hospital, knowing that I'd "had it". How's that for a coincidence? It's quite unintentional, the architects chose the twenty-second.'

After a lengthy silence she whispered, 'Pat, it's uncanny, isn't it?'

I smiled . . . uncanny? Yes or maybe that 'Someone' planned it that way.

A foundation-stone laying ceremony . . . who to ask? Professor Easson, Director of Radiotherapy, should be asked to 'chair' the proceedings. Then, of course, Sir William Downward and those members of the Central Committee who could come. The Branches of the Fund? It would be marvellous if all of them could be there, but if any *one* of them should be asked to represent them all, who better than Paddy Hayward, whose late, courageous wife Julé had made such a magnificent contribution? Then there were our Patrons, Sir Matt Busby and Ken Dodd. I would like them to come, not only because of their own efforts but also to represent all that the worlds of Sport and Show Business had done to help the Fund. And what about the thousands and thousands of ordinary men, women and children who had provided the bulk of the money that made all this possible. I'd like to stretch out my arms and encompass them all . . . an elderly person and a child . . . that would be symbolic of the entire age range.

Oh, Doctor Hounsfield, what a lot of hard work your invention has caused us!

It would be wonderful if he could be there when that stone was laid. Would he come? These scientists travel the world, lecturing to people in their own field . . . he could be in Vancouver, Tokyo, Toronto or Timbuktu for all I knew.

Ring and find out! If you don't ask, you'll never know!

I did, and Doctor Godfrey Hounsfield said that he'd be delighted to come.

That put the seal on it, for me.

Had we known it, we couldn't have picked a worse day. The weather was freezingly cold; the national news was a catalogue of doom, gloom and despondency and 22nd January was the date chosen for one-day token strikes by members of several trade unions. By the time we knew of this, plans for the laying of the foundation stone were more or less complete, so we decided to go ahead with them, come what may.

Biting winds, a grey and overcast sky with the occasional flurry of snowflakes, yet *nothing* could have taken the sunshine out of that day for me. My emotions ran high. Elation, a sense of achievement and also one of incredulity for it was a day I hadn't expected to see.

Professor Eric Easson welcomed the guests and said that the medical team at the Christie were impatient to have and to use the scanner, with all the advantages it offered to patients and because of the valuable research it would initiate.

'We will, I am sure, be able to cure more patients than in the past. It will allow us to plan our treatment with radiation in a more accurate and precise way. The sooner it is installed, the better.'

One of my favourite people, Bobby Charlton, deputised for Sir Matt Busby, who was in London. Ken Dodd, our other Patron, spent most of the morning trying to get his car started and couldn't be with us, which was disappointing both for Ken and for us.

I thanked Sir William Downward for all the work the Central Committee had done to steer the project successfully to this memorable day. I asked Mr Hayward to accept my thanks on behalf of the branches of the Fund who had worked so hard in support of me.

Then came the laying of the stone.

Beside me were ten-year-old Nicola Farrow, a schoolmate of the late little Jane Butler of Acacias County Primary School and eighty-four-year-old Mrs Olive Snowdon of Blackpool, a pensioner who had supported the Fund since its inception. It would have been marvellous if I could have had with me all the many thousands of people who had helped me, but that would need something about the size of Wembley Stadium.

Instead, they were represented by Olive and Nicola, who each put a trowelful of mortar under the stone. Then, I put my trowel of mortar there, the stone was positioned and we tapped it into place with a gavel.

'Come on, Doctor Hounsfield, you started all this. *You* help lay this stone, too,' I invited.

There we were, four happy, smiling people – and the job was done. Attending as my personal guests were Kay Fisher and Beryl Acton, my lifelong friends, and Sister Marie Calvert, my ministering angel and District Nurse. Patients, watching from the windows above the old entrance hall, cheered.

When the ceremony was over, there was Vera, the auxiliary nurse who'd comforted me on that day, two years ago, when I'd been told I'd 'had it'. Now, her face was wreathed in smiles.

'We've done it, Pat! We've done it!'

As I walked towards her, I held out my arms. We hugged each other and how I managed *not* to burst into tears, I'll never know. I thought of Flo Wilson, of Julé Hayward, of Roger Shires, treasurer of the Poulton Branch, who'd died in November . . . all of them cancer patients who had worked so hard and who hadn't lived to see this day . . . or had they? Yes, I believe they would know.

As Geoff and I left the Christie by the main entrance, more patients lined the windows of the wards at the front of the hospital. They waved and cheered and wished me well.

'One step nearer!' I called to them.

They say the Press are a hard lot. Maybe we are when we're chasing a story and maybe I've applied a similar tenacity to this Appeal. Off the job, we're like any other people, for many journalists and photographers have experienced the cancer problem within their own families. The help they have given me has been invaluable. Without them, I could not have let the need be known and if I'd added up all the column inches written about the Appeal and had to pay for them as advertising space, it would have taken every penny we've raised.

It was only when we got home later in the afternoon that I realised that I hadn't seen the *front* of that foundation stone, or read the inscription. I had to wait for the BBC regional news on 'Look North' to get my first glimpse of it.

It stated, simply: 'This stone was laid by Patricia Seed, MBE on 22nd January 1979'. It seemed to me that stone recorded not only my name, but my heart and soul.

As the news item ended, presenter Stuart Hall said: 'Yes . . . thirty of my ties and twelve of my cookbooks have gone into that Fund of yours, love!'

I went to Garstang the following morning and bought Stuart the gaudiest tie I could find. I sent it to him with a note: 'Have this one on me – not only to help replace part of your sadly depleted wardrobe, but also as a token of my thanks to my pals of "Look North" for their invaluable help.' After all, 'Look North' had recorded the first steps of the journey. They'd been in on it from the very beginning.

There is no way, now, short of an earthquake or some equally horrid, unforeseen disaster, that the Christie will not have that scanner. I hope I am there on that day next autumn when the Department of Computerised Axial Tomography is officially opened and that first patient is scanned. The chances are that for once in my life I will be speechless, standing there with tears streaming down my face. I remember a television interviewer asking me if I thought I'd be there on that day. I remember my reply: 'I certainly hope so, but if I'm not there in person, I'll be there in spirit.'

We have to play whatever hand fate deals to us. In the last couple of years or so, I have been dealt two hands. I haven't played either of them close to my chest. They've been played uppermost on the table, in the full view of anyone who cared to see. The first hand, a single card whose name is Cancer. A bitter fury against the disease, which, I was told, was going to mean 'curtains' for me and separate me from those I loved, made me want to hit back. The how, the why and the where have already been chronicled in these pages.

Pauline has talked about coincidences . . . is it just coincidence that when I first went into the Christie in May 1976, my photographer son should show me pictures and an article about the CAT scanner? *Was* it coincidence? Or was it Destiny, Fate, Providence or the guiding hand of an Almighty Being who uses us mortal creatures for his purpose? 'Put yourself in His hands . . . you are merely a tool . . .' The reader must draw his own conclusions. There are no doubts in my mind.

In trying to fight back in a practical, constructive way, fate dealt me a second hand. This time, the full suit of hearts and three aces. The full suit of hearts? Little children, octogenarians and all age groups in between. Thousands upon thousands of people who have seen fit to join in the fight, giving of their best with such an unparalleled goodwill and to such an extent that one is left wondering where the human race goes wrong. Their response has by-passed or ignored social status, age, sex, race, creed, colour and political affiliations. It has united some of the highest families in the land with some of its humblest citizens. They have devoted their time, their talents and their energy; they have used initiative, imagination and ingenuity in honest endeavour for the benefit of future patients of this world-renowned hospital.

I think it was David Garrick who said: 'A fellow feeling makes one wondrous kind.' That new department will be a testimony to a caring society. Every brick, every stone, every nut, bolt and screw will only be there because so very many people have cared sufficiently to make it so.

And the three aces? Faith, Hope, Charity. My faith that people would respond. This they have done, unstintingly. In doing so, they have provided new hope, a lifeline for many north-west cancer patients, and it's all been accomplished in the name of charity, the other word for which is Love.

What has all this meant to me? Maybe I'm luckier than most people who get this disease in that I *know* now, why I had to have it. Whatever the personal outcome, I know that I have not had cancer for nothing. Behind all things, there is a reason even it at times it escapes us, or is obscured.

I admit that it has been hard work and there is no doubt at all that it has proved excellent therapy for me. I remember my dear grandmother used to say: 'Hard work never killed anybody, but the thought of it kills some folk.' There have been nights when I didn't want to leave my armchair and a warm fireside to set out in cold wet winter conditions to attend an event in some distant town or village; when I didn't want to answer the phone; when the thought of the mountains of mail to be answered daunted me; when I'd crave for leisure time to join in with whatever my family were doing, or spend an evening with my friends. I do not regret any of it. I have always been glad that I have been able to share in some of the effort which has taken place. Some 25,000 miles of travelling along the 'Scanner Trail' has taken me to bingo halls and baronial halls; to clubs, pubs, offices, shops, factories, churches and schools to meet people who were working equally as hard as I, in support of this project. My regret is that it has been a physical impossibility to meet everyone who has contributed to this achievement. There have been quite a few tears and some headaches along the way, but the 'Scanner Trail' has brought me an abundance of love, comradeship and laughter.

Adjectives such as 'brave', 'courageous' and even 'national heroine' have been used and there have been those who have asked me, 'What's it like to be famous?' To be honest, I don't think of myself as any of these things. I am still 'Mrs Average' – a wife and a mother. Now, there's the added bonus of being grandmother to Helen's daughter, the sweetest little baby girl. She's called Victoria after me. She's the apple of my eye and the grandchild I thought I'd never live to see. As far as I am concerned, I am just an ordinary woman, who, through circumstances not of her own making, found herself in a place, at a time, with the qualifications necessary to be able to meet a need. And yet, I know that life can never be quite the same again. How could it be? The 'Scanner Trail' has widened my horizons, broadened my experience. In pursuit of the Appeal, I have met people I would never have met in other circumstances; Royal people, rich people; famous people of the stage, stars of the big and the small screen and radio; sporting personalities and even the most famous racehorse of all time. I have met men, women and children of every walk of life and as a result, I have very many good and loyal friends I would not otherwise have known. They have made the 'Scanner Trail' a truly rewarding and enriching experience. Money can be counted. Machinery can be made to do its work. No price could be placed upon the undiluted generosity of spirit which I have been privileged to witness and to share. I thank God for it.

In recent months, a lot of accolades have come my way. I appreciate that they are recognition of the job I have tried to do. Sometimes, when I'm in my kitchen doing mundane, routine chores, such as washing the dishes or peeling the vegetables, my mind runs free and I wonder, did these things really happen? There have been the big occasions. Big, that is, as far as prestige and stature goes. But much as I value and am proud of my silver medal in its leather case, I value equally other awards. For instance, the illuminated plaque given to me by an eighty-three-year-old lady from Wigan. It took a lot of effort for old Miss Laign to make this gift. She has suffered three strokes, has difficulty in walking and her right hand and arm are paralysed. Holding her pens and brushes in her right hand and steadying it by gripping her right wrist with her left hand, it took her ten minutes to complete each single letter of the following:

God give me the SERENITY to accept the
    things I cannot change.
The COURAGE to change the things I can
And the WISDOM to know the difference.

What *price* does one put on that or on the love which went
into its making? Similarly, I recall the young mother in
Burnley who with her two-year-old daughter in her arms,
handed me a single carnation wrapped in florist's paper with
the words, 'Thank you for bringing out the best in us all.' The
flower eventually withered and died. The memory of it will
live for ever in my mind and in my heart. I remember also
the young housewives in Barrowford, no longer isolated in
their homes but now a community where friendship is
paramount.

These things are riches beyond the dreams of avarice and the
common denominator is Love. The poorest human being has
as much of it to give as the richest man on earth. All it costs
any of us is ourselves and how much of ourselves we are prepared to give away. If, because I love my own family so
dearly, it prompted me to do this work for love of other
people, that love has been returned to me a thousandfold.

No woman could ask for greater reward and these are the
personal riches I have found along the 'Scanner Trail'. And
what has it all cost me? What is the price I have had to pay?
There is the time I might have spent with my family, but none
of us have any regrets about that. Professionally, it is in-
hibiting in that a humorous or pungent article on any other
subject might cause surprise or create the wrong image.

'And what are you going to do next? Where do you go
from here?'

Naturally, I'd like to devote more of my time to my family
and in the last two years I've had little opportunity to follow
my own profession. On the other hand, I know that I wouldn't
have time for anything at all, but for the expertise of the

Christie. That hospital is in need of many things. To name but two, the Outpatients Department requires modernising and extending; one of the first things to be axed under the Government's cut-back in spending was the updating of the X-ray Diagnostics Department which at present is like a rabbit warren, where – to their credit – the staff manage to provide an efficient facility under extremely difficult and archaic conditions. To my mind, *these* things should be funded from government sources. However, one has to face that fact that technology never stands still and for much of it there will be no government money forthcoming. Within the next couple of years or so, some of the technologies at present being researched will become marketable products and some are already of great interest to those involved in cancer medicine and treatment. It would be nice to have something in the kitty the next time around and put that second storey above the new CAT Department. For that reason, the Appeal will continue, for the sake of cancer patients of the future.

Meanwhile, much needs to be done in furtherance of Cancer Education. There is a need to constantly chip away at the misconceptions and confusion that the word provokes. Hardest of all to reach are those who deliberately 'switch off' when the word is mentioned. They just don't want to know. Yet if one were to suggest that they plunge across a busy highway with their eyes closed in the hope that by so doing, the traffic would disappear and they'd reach the other pavement in safety, they'd say one was mad. 'Don't be daft,' they'd reply, 'without getting a phobia about it, we're alert to the dangers, and have regard for the traffic signals.'

What is so different about adopting the same attitude to cancer? Surely it is better to be aware of the danger, to have regard for the signals and if in any doubt at all, to seek advice, rather than live – or possibly die – in the hope that by shutting one's eyes, IT WILL NOT HAPPEN TO YOU. Statistics tell us how many people are killed on the roads each year. They *don't* tell us how many people used the road in safety, because they applied some common sense. With a bit of sound common sense, many of the dangers of cancer could be averted or treated. Observing the signals could significantly increase the cure rate

During the course of the Appeal, many cancer patients and relatives have written to me. Some cancer patients have telephoned, sometimes talking for an hour or more, pouring out their worries and fears to me in the knowledge that they were talking to someone who would understand. Some of these men and women have been at their wits' end. Is there a need for an organisation especially geared to help them? Such a scheme would need a great deal of preparatory groundwork before it was launched on a regional or national basis and to be avoided like the plague would be an organisation which degenerated into pathetic, maudlin little groups where people swopped symptoms, tried to out-do each other in tales of suffering, or beefed about their doctors or the local hospital. A sympathetic understanding and a kindly practicality would be the keynotes. Counsellors would need to know where every kind of help was available, from domestic home-help to terminal nursing care. One thing they would not do is offer medical advice. Only doctors and consultants can give that.

This is something about which I am 'doing my homework' at present. For once committed, I am incapable of half measures and that is the reason why I am not precipitating myself into premature action. If there is a guiding hand, no doubt I will be pointed in the right direction when the time is appropriate. Meanwhile, the first task has yet to be completed. We have not yet reached the end of the 'Scanner Trail'.

As I write, the Fund has just topped the one and a half million pounds but there is still some way to go. This figure includes over £72,000 of interest and we have used less than £8,000 to administer the Fund, the bulk of which has been spent on postage. As a charity, I would think those figures make it unique, but then, I was never much good at mathematics. On the home front, there is thankfulness that Geoff and I are still together. For how long, we do not know. Without him, I know that I could not have initiated this Appeal. He has been the rock upon whom I have leaned, the man to whom I have turned for encouragement, advice, solace and whose patient understanding has supported me along the entire length of the 'Trail'. We have love, respect, friendship and truly a partnership.

Maybe, in January 1982, the Christie will give me the 'five years cancer free' clearance, in which case, the prayers and good wishes of many will have been answered. (That's when I've promised myself I'll give up smoking cigarettes.) Meanwhile, the recipe is the same – one day at a time. In the autumn, there is much to look forward to. My Cnetral Committee and I are hopeful that Her Royal Highness will find it possible to accept our invitation to open the new department. Personally, I would be delighted and very proud if t³e Duchess finds this can be fitted into her engagement diary. Not only because she is a member of our Royal Family, but also because she is a Northern lass and it would set the seal on the tremendous efforts made by so many other Northern lasses to make the project a reality. My globe-trotting friend Tess Pickford returns from the Solomon Islands. Her recent letter tells me of the almost unbearable heat in the Solomons and she says how much she is looking forward to an English winter. In the snow-ridden depths of January, I have my own thoughts on that, none of which are printable! But I have no doubt we shall have tales to tell each other, stories to relate, which will take us a month of Sundays to get through. As most good friends do we will probably just pick up where we left off and like an old, comfortable pair of shoes, retrace the miles we've travelled. In conclusion, my mind takes me back to a day just over one month ago, Christmas Day, 1978.

My family and I were gathered around our dining table (*still* with that small drill hole), and there was warmth, laughter and happiness. On the table was the turkey and the trimmings. Three generations of us, six happy smiling faces; Geoff and me, our son Mike, our daughter Helen and her husband Gerard and, in her high chair, too small to know what it was all about, our adorable little Victoria. Her inseparable companion, Bonnie Boy, was sitting on the floor, strategically positioned near to her, ready to retrieve anything which might fall his way.

My beloved family . . . my greatest blessing and my inspiration. Had I not loved them so much, the 'Scanner Trail' would never have begun. We raised our glasses and wished each other a 'Happy Christmas' and then toasted 'absent friends'. I included all the people who had journeyed along the 'Trail' with me. We pulled our Christmas crackers and searched among the torn crêpe paper for the fancy hats, the plastic toys, the mottoes. Mine said: Miracles CAN happen, but one has to work terribly hard to make them happen.

Another coincidence, Pauline?

Later, like many other families throughout the country and the Commonwealth, we listened to the Queen's Christmas message and heard the recording of her father, King George VI, quote those immortal lines:

'I said to the Man who stood at the gate of the year, "Give me a light that I may tread safely into the unknown," and he replied, "Go out into the darkness and put your hand into the hand of God. That shall be unto you better than a light and safer than a known way." '

In place of fear, I had put my hand trustingly and without sanctimony into his. I had trod the path along which he chose to lead me.

I had seen how miracles happened.

All you need is Love.

Index

287